BAREFOOT DOCTOR'S HANDBOOK FOR MODERN LOVERS

BAREFOOT DOCTOR'S HANDBOOKFOR MODERNLOVERS

a **Spiritual Guide** to Truly Amazing **LOVE** and **sex**

BROADWAY BOOKS • NEW YORK

BROADWAY

This book was originally published in 2000 in Great Britain by Judy Piatkus
(Publishers) Ltd.

Visit our website at www.broadwaybooks.com

Library of Congress Cataloging-in-Publication Data

Russell, Stephen, 1954–
Barefoot doctor's handbook for modern lovers: a spiritual
guide to truly amazing love and sex / Stephen Russell.—1st ed.
p.   cm.
1. Sex. 2. Love. 3. Tao. I. Title.
HQ31 .R934 2001
306.7—dc21   00-050789

First Edition in the United States of America

Designed by Bonni Leon-Berman
Illustrated by Bill Reid

ISBN 0-7679-0700-0
10 9 8 7 6 5 4 3 2 1

Supportive Quotation

"THIS IS A FUCKING CLASSIC."
J. Catto

I dedicate this with love
to K.—you've got to be clever
to keep it going forever—C.,
and to all young lovers
wherever you are.

CONTENTS

Author's Wayward Foreword   *xvii*

THE SETUP (the seduction)   1
Warning and disclaimer   3
"Love-sexy"   4
Don't be fooled by the experts (author's credentials)   5
Hello from/confessions of a barefoot doctor   6
So what's the angle?   8
Why would you need a handbook about it?   9
This is a handbook for *all* modern lovers (and that means you)   10
Shout going out to all the women in the house (sisters)   11
Shout going out to all the boys   11
Shout going out to all the gay men   12
Shout going out to all the lesbians   12
Shout going out to all the pervs, s 'n' m freaks, auto-eroticists,
    fetishists, and other assorted deviant adventurers   13
Shout going out to all the old bastards (and dears)   13
And if there're any first-timers out there tonight . . .   14
What *is* a modern lover?   14
The story of "O"   17
Use of the vernacular   17
My own personal motivations for presenting this material (in
    case you want to know)   18
How to take optimum advantage of the text   20
Wayward Taoist philosophical premises and morals (as if)   20
Sex as a spiritual path   22

The Tao 24
The universe is consciousness made manifest 25
Yin and Yang 26
Chi 27
Balance 28
Love 29
Sexual love 30
Recreational sex vs. procreational sex 30
Beauty 31
All girls and boys are spiritual sisters and brothers, hence
  sex is incest on a grand scale 32
All beings, at their roots, are one, hence sex is just the Tao
  jerking off 32
Sex and connecting with the mystery of creation 33
You're free to do whatever you choose 34
Not necessarily good, not necessarily bad 34
The nonsense of morals 35
Relationships, the illusion of 37
Being/feeling sexy 38
Making yourself feel/look attractive 40
Vanity/self-consciousness 41
Hygiene 41
Smells/scents 42
Props/setting 43
Stop performing and start feeling 43
Enacting the eternal dance of Yin and Yang 44
More love 46
The Three Tan Tiens 46
Sharing consciousness 49
Eroticism 50
Acting out vs. containment 52

Contents ✛   xi

The nature of desire   53
The nature of passion   55
The nature of pure sexual intelligence vs. fantasy   56
The significance of smell   59
Importance of being comfortable with your own sexuality   60
Self-esteem   61
Inhibitions   63
Being rude   63
Importance of physical fitness, flexibility, suppleness, and stamina   64
Taking your clothes off   64
The significance of movement   66
Sexual nirvana   67
Tempo   68
Alertness to signals   69
Counting repetitions as meditation   70
No longer needing to distract yourself with ugly thoughts to
    prevent premature ejaculation   70
The question of premature ejaculation   71
The mystery of chemistry   73
Dynamics   74
Are there such things as soul mates?   75
Moments, series of   75
Is there a perfect mate?   76
Dropping expectations   76
The case for serial monogamy   77
It's all just a play in the mind   79
The case for nonserial monogamy   80
The case for the floating harem   81
Importance of flirting   82
Nature of seduction   84
Boundaries and personal/interpersonal space   85

Trust　　　　　　　　　　　　　　　　　　　　　85

Communication　　　　　　　　　　　　　　　86

Honesty　　　　　　　　　　　　　　　　　　　88

Honesty as an aphrodisiac　　　　　　　　　　89

Dishonesty　　　　　　　　　　　　　　　　　89

Is my dick too small?　　　　　　　　　　　　90

Dishonesty as an aphrodisiac　　　　　　　　91

Everyone's responsible for their own experience here　92

Manners, discretion, and confidentiality　　　92

Falling in love　　　　　　　　　　　　　　　93

Integrity/lack of　　　　　　　　　　　　　　95

Fidelity　　　　　　　　　　　　　　　　　　96

Loyalty　　　　　　　　　　　　　　　　　　97

Treachery　　　　　　　　　　　　　　　　　97

Deceit　　　　　　　　　　　　　　　　　　　99

Lying/denying　　　　　　　　　　　　　　　100

All is fair in love and war　　　　　　　　　101

Being friends　　　　　　　　　　　　　　　102

Commitment　　　　　　　　　　　　　　　　103

Sex with strangers in confined spaces　　　　103

The vast importance of condoms　　　　　　104

Turning your whole body into an erogenous zone　107

Feigning/exaggerating pleasure/faking an orgasm　109

More on the importance of physical fitness, flexibility,
　　suppleness, and stamina　　　　　　　　　110

Intensification of sexual tension　　　　　　111

Breathing　　　　　　　　　　　　　　　　　112

Slowing the breath tempo　　　　　　　　　112

Breathing together (with O)　　　　　　　　113

Fancy postures　　　　　　　　　　　　　　114

Relaxation　　　　　　　　　　　　　　　　115

Four ounces   116
The Big Squeeze   117
The question of orgasms   121
Use your voice (to talk/moan) during sex   122
Inner alchemy   124
Cold sex vs. warm sex   127
Planning the moment vs. letting the moment happen   128
Acting out fantasies   129
The question of masturbation   129
The question of sperm retention   131
Dirty, what's dirty?   133
Eyes open vs. eyes closed   133
Stopping when you want   134
Stopping the internal commentary   136
The techniques and you   138
The perfect fuck   139
So what?   141
'Nuff seduction?   141

THE STING (what you actually do)   143
Reminder   145
Gateway to the Soul in the sole   145
Supporting the jade pillow   146
Wind in the willows   146
Small golden apple   148
Calves   149
Behind the knees   149
Knuckles   150
Between the fingers   151
Elbow creases   151
Base of the spine   152

Sucking/licking between toes   152
Using your toes   153
Inside ankles   153
Toe in the Hole   154
Heart-to-heart connection   154
Pubic pinch   155
Zygomatic kisses   155
Sucking nipple   156
Worshiping ass   159
The French kiss   162
Hand jobs   164
O-girl, manual clitoral stimulation thereof   168
Meeting belly   170
Blow jobs   171
Cunnilingus, the joys of   174
Soixante-neuf   177
Putting two fingers up   178
Scratching   179
Biting   180
Pinching   181
Tickling   182
Fucking, positions thereof   183
Moving gracefully between positions   185
Sacred entry   187
Shallow thrust   188
Medium thrust   188
Full thrust   189
Mixing up your thrusts   189
Riding the shudders   190
The Sexual Stillpoint   191
Full-power pumping   191

Contents ✛   XV

Alternating rhythms	192
Fucking O in the ass	193
Grinding	194
Augmenting coital stimulation with hand/foot/mouth action	194
Transcendental aspect	195
Connecting your Three (Six) Tan Tiens	197
Whooshing the Chi	199
Effective postorgasmic phase management	202

THE PAYOFF (postorgasmic blatherings)	**205**
What about sexual problems?	207
Rape	208
Complexes	209
Frigidity	210
Vaginismus	210
Impotence	211
Nervous willy	211
Sexually transmitted diseases (STDs)	213
Unwanted pregnancy	214
Sudden Surprise Ejaculation Syndrome (SSES)	215
Inability to orgasm	216
Sadomasochism, bondage, marriage, and other perversions	216
Prostitution	218
Threesomes/fivesomes/sevensomes/orgies	219
Sex parties	221
Perversion	221
The problem of incest	222
The problem of child abuse	223
Sex toys	225
Lubricants	226
Aphrodisiacs	226

Alcohol and sex 227
Drugs and sex 227
The problem of sexual possessiveness 228
Pornography as a stimulant 229
Cozy/lazy vs. sexy 229
Using sex as a distraction 231
Using sex as a form of stress relief 231
The problem of fluctuating libido levels 231
Celibacy 232
Always be prepared 232
Using sex as a substitute for human warmth 232
Sex with strangers vs. sex with your mate 233
Sex with friends 233
The problem of promiscuity/sex addiction 233
Pregnancy and sex 234
Sex in the nine months or so after pregnancy 234
Marriage and sex 234
Divorce and sex 234
Age differences 234
Living with the moon 235
Wishing on an orgasm (white magic) 236
Avoiding the pitfalls of practicing alone and falling in love
with yourself 237
Cyber-sex 237
The perils of prolonged wind retention and other gross matters 238
The nonsense of breaking people's hearts 238
How to avoid unnecessary aggravation 239
Taking one's leave graciously 239

THANK-YOUS 241
Index 247

AUTHOR'S WAYWARD foreword

Barefoot Doctor's Handbook for Modern Lovers, A Spiritual Guide to Truly Amazing Love and Sex does just that: provides a Wayward Taoist guide to help you discover new depths of sexual love within yourself.

I have come (fairly) clean in this book about my own sexuality in the hope that modern lovers the world over will be inspired to do likewise, as I believe that bringing things out into the open is good for people's health and will be helpful in reducing general tension levels on the planet at this time. Moreover, it will hopefully make for some interesting and enjoyable theater.

I present the following material, not to shock or show off in any way, but to share with you, humbly and honestly, the vast wealth of sexual experience I have gained, both as a professional healer and private aficionado, as it would be a shame to let it go unwritten.

In so doing, I write as I would speak to you if I were in the room with you now (and I wasn't trying to behave myself and watch my language because you were the queen/king or someone of similar standing). As a result, words often considered taboo pop up in the text with some frequency, as do instances of inevitable schoolboy humor, alongside descriptions of extreme explicitness. For this reason, you may find it expedient to keep this handbook far from the hands of children or be prepared for some pretty frank discussion.

THE**SETUP**
(the seduction)

Warning and disclaimer

be warned: what follows is potentially subversive, may result in untimely death, and furthermore is written by a rogue with the morals of an alley cat.

(Hidden within its secret folds) this handbook contains the key to sexual love. Sexual love is a very dangerous thing. Once you start messing around with it, you are inviting powerful forces into the cracks in your daily schedule which can severely derange you, often permanently.

Reading the following material and practicing the methods suggested can radically alter your fundamental socio-sexual behavioral patterns. This constitutes an experiment with reality, the results of which cannot possibly be predicted.

An unsettling period of sexual disorientation may occur before you reach the herewith promised state of sexual nirvana, if indeed you do.

It is impossible/impractical to universalize sexual advice. Everyone responds to information differently. Everyone responds to sex differently (with different people at different times). Consequently, the material is open to misinterpretation and subsequent faulty sexual practices may result. It's not without the realms of possibility in this instance that you may variously lose complete sexual interest and enter holy orders, become a wanton slut/

libertine, switch from straight to gay or vice versa, wreck your marriage/long-term relationship, give up a life of freedom to get married, or catch something and die young.

If you do manifest any development not to your liking, i.e., if your whole life gets fucked up as a result of playing with this material, neither I, the publishers, nor anyone involved in the global production and marketing of this book will be held legally or morally responsible in any way.

That notwithstanding, my belief (and wish) is that reading this handbook will greatly enhance the value and increase the frequency of quality sexual experience in your life, thereby making you a happier, healthier person, who's far more sexually confident and fun to be around and who consequently gets laid more often (and that you'll be singing "Barefoot Doctor is a brick" from the rooftops).

"Love-sexy"

This material concerns one expression of love, perhaps the most momentarily intense. It's been around since the start of things, yet no one seems to have grown bored with it, indeed it has never failed to rivet the attention (from time to time) of even the most abstract of thinkers: sex with other people. Or to be more precise, expressing sexual love with other people.

Sex as an expression of anything other than love is like food without nutritional value. It fills the gap for an instant, then you're hungry again. Sex as an expression of love nourishes you in a cumulative way, each encounter building your sense of self-value, increasing your capacity to love yourself and others.

Not that there's anything intrinsically wrong (or right) with loveless sex. Fast food is sometimes the expedient choice. Fast sex can be exhilarating. But just as your digestive organs find it hard to make much use of mass-market burgers, your soul finds it hard to make sense of loveless sexual encounters.

You don't need to be in a long-term relationship to express love when you have sex. You can express love with a complete stranger as easily as you can express no love with a long-term partner. That part's entirely up to you.

Credit to The Artist for coining the phrase "love-sexy." This is a handbook on the mechanics of accessing, developing, and refining love-sexy to the utmost spiritual degree (and making it work in your busy schedule).

Don't be fooled by the experts
(author's credentials)

Barefoot doctor has been schooled in the Taoist art of love and sex (Taoist sexology) by more than one great master/mistress, and has devoted many thousands of hours to real-time practicing, refining, perfecting, and generally engaging in practical (hands-on) research. (This is not to suggest Barefoot Doctor's a sex maniac or social deviant. Just a reasonably good-looking, single [for now], heterosexual guy in his early/mid-forties with a fairly good sense of humor, a healthy sex drive/curiosity, and hell, things happen.)

He has written a previous international best-seller on the Taoist art of sexual massage, and as well as his "regular" healing work, has practiced as a sexual therapist with thousands of individuals in both private treatment and workshop scenarios over the twenty-one years he's been in practice. However, these factors notwithstanding, he feels it foolhardy to claim anything as grandiose as expertise, or to present from such a standpoint.

For with all that "knowledge," practice, and experimentation, both personal and professional, I still suffer (would you believe) variously, from time to time, with Nervous Willy (dick), so-called premature/surprise ejaculation, lack of interest, inaccurate clitoris-locating skills, insensitivity, clumsiness, laziness, general physical insecurities, and even "adolescent" complexes about penis girth and length. (General consensus is it's a happy medium, unless they were *all* being polite.)

Hence, far be it from me to come on like some "big" sex expert who's talking down to you, the mortal reader. No, I'm as sexually flawed and fucked up as the next barefoot doctor.

I experience the same shit as everyone else, i.e., you, but through practicing the Taoist art of (love and) sex have learned to turn that shit to my advantage (and therefore to the advantage of those with whom I share the sexual experience, i.e., fuck).

So I'm sharing this handbook as one confused modern lover with another (everyone is, believe me), so that you can take advantage of these ancient yet not crusty, indeed, extremely excellent, Taoist sexual secrets, too.

Hello from/confessions of a barefoot doctor

The rich and varied sexual episodes that have occurred for me around this merry globe have, overall, been of supreme enjoyment to both myself and, as far as shown, to those who also took part. They have also provided me (and I hope them) with an infinite stream of intriguing living-theater, personal development/education, and spiritual growth.

As for orientation, I am a confirmed/semicompulsive hetero-sexual (I *love* women), have served a total of eleven years' marriage with two different (very strong) women, have three sons, two of whom are bigger and taller than me (and I ain't no shrimp) and all three of whom are far more handsome, whom I love to beyond eternity. At the time of writing (this page) I am totally free and un-encumbered by contract, obligation, or simple agreement to up-hold an exclusive situation with any one woman, and am having a *fucking ball.*

However, owing to the alchemical process of writing this book and the effects of that upon my personal life, synchronized with the effects of the astrological warps and flutters of the planets in my chart, I have a deep-felt intuition that this situation could do an easy one-eighty any time now, so I'm rejoicing in how it is now and hope some of that joy rubs off on you.

While maintaining full empathetic appreciation of the homo-sexual experience (whatever blows your hair back, baby), my per-sonal preference is for women. I love them. In all shapes and sizes (within certain parameters). I love the sensual essence of woman as much as I love my own. For in that essence I touch divinity.

Call me Renegade Taoist Womanizer (RTW), many do (mis-takenly of course), but I hold that sharing the mystery of the sex-ual moment is one of the most joyous and life-enhancing acts of spiritual service a person can perform/engage in, and I personally am grateful to have been given those opportunities to serve (it's an honor).

I pray this equips me adequately to now serve in this, the hum-ble way of the simple handbook writer, and that with every orgasm you enjoy henceforth, the angels sing hallelujah.

I write then, not as an expert (I don't believe there is such a thing), but as a (still) curious, enthusiastic, fascinated, sometimes bumbling and incompetent mortal, who's learned enough old Taoist sex tricks to (know better and) be able to pass on something of value. And furthermore to entertain you with the wry, "unauthodox" angle of a modern, Wayward Taoist slut.

I have no morals (I am amoral), save for the one that says do whatever you do with kindness, love if you can manage it, and respect for all life.

So what's the angle?

Spiritualizing your sex.

Meaning?

Sex is not about bodies. Sex is about consciousness. As with all Taoist methods, Wayward or otherwise, you reframe your experience of sex action by shifting your perspective. What happens then is the opposite of a mindless shag and radically different from a sexual performance.

The so-called sexual arena—bed/floor/kitchen table/office desk, etc.—becomes transformed, of itself, into a primordial temple of life/spirit, by refining the sexual pulse/flow until it becomes pure chi/superhuman energy. Once you have this chi at your disposal, you can then intensify it exponentially by whooshing it around each other's bodies in an inner dance of spirit(s) leading to that stratum of reality known as immortality, which is completely indescribable, so I'll stop now. [See *Whooshing the Chi*, p. 199.]

When this dance kicks off for real, your spirits enter the highest state of pure nothingness (Wu Chi) and you are at liberty to enter the heavenly realms of sexual nirvana. [See *Sexual nirvana*, p. 67.] This equates to the biggest orgasm you can ever imagine filling your entire being, all the way from the tips of your toes to the crown of your head, sustaining itself in the ebb and flow of an endless tide of cosmic pleasure, wave upon wave of it lapping against your shore.

You like that shit?

Well, I'd rather you got a little more down to earth about it. (I'm willing to go with you on this spiritual sex tip, but I've got to understand what you're talking about, Doc.)

Spiritualizing your sex means turning your sex into your meditation. We all know the benefits of meditation—you become more peaceful, more focused, more clear-thinking, more electric, for you and your partner(s). In other words, you stand a chance of becoming enlightened by practicing what you most enjoy: a damn good fuck.

I get that (thank you).

It's OK, and I could keep waffling around this thought-circle saying nothing, but if you'd care to set about picking up some of this for yourself, tarry here no longer and read on.

Why would you need a handbook about it?

You don't need one. You may *want* one, however, for one of the following reasons:

- You've just met a new lover and want to impress him/her.
- You're in training. (You want to impress the next new lover you meet.)
- Sex with your current lover/long-term partner has grown stale and you want to spark things up.
- You've become aware of your sexual inadequacies and it irks you because you wish to be perfect.
- You wish to impress others with the vaguely experimental/quasi-spiritual nature of the contents of your bookshelf.

- You're a perv.
- You fancy a new text to flick through on the toilet.
- You're suffering from Prevailing Endemic Sexual Confusion (PESC) and want to make things even more difficult for yourself.
- You fancy yourself as sexual superwoman/man/both and will take any handy hints you can get.
- You need a new pillow for your Alexander yoga sessions.
- Plain old curiosity (about sex/barefoot doctors).
- You simply want to be entertained.

This is a handbook for *all* modern lovers
(and that means you)

Regardless of your age, gender, orientation, strange preferences, weird habits, religious/spiritual persuasion, marital/relationship status, or any other obstacles you may care to imagine, this handbook is written for you.

Whether you're not getting enough, getting too much, getting the wrong kind, in renunciation/celibacy (voluntary or otherwise), sex-addicted, frigid, impotent, underage, overage, totally dysfunctional, totally got it licked, or whatever you can think of, everyone, one way or another, has an issue of some kind, to some extent, at various times, with finding full, satisfactory expression of the primal sexual urge on a sustainable, life-enhancing basis.

Whatever role you're currently playing in the primordial melodrama, the psychosexual perception-shifting "exercises" and somatic pleasure-enhancing techniques presented in this text are intended to expand your current sphere of sexual activity and may, if practiced correctly, provide you with a new slant on all aspects of your daily life, not just the sex bits.

Shout going out to all
the women in the house
(sisters)

Bear with me. As hard as I try otherwise, I can only write from a male perspective. I cannot speak from your sexual viewpoint without becoming one of you. Which I've sometimes longed to do, at least for an afternoon/evening or two, just so I could indulge in the evident pleasures of lesbian love, and also go on a girls' night out.

But though I've paid consistent attention to developing the female (Yin) energies within me along with the male (Yang), I now accept that this unrequitable fantasy will not be realized in this lifetime, no matter how much meditational/inner-alchemical hocus-pocus I get up to.

No matter. This material is written as expressly for you as it is for the boys. So make allowances for my male perspective being the exact opposite of your own, and take unto thy breast all the information on offer herein without gender qualms.

Shout going out to
all the boys

This can be a tricky business, one man playing the role of sexual adviser to another. For however evolved we become, we never seem very far from reacting like wild animals toward each other, plugging in to that primal layer of our being where we compete with one another, as in who of us here is the biggest, fastest, strongest, most sexually accomplished and handsome.

I saw through that competition illusion a while back, when it finally clicked that we're not competitors, we're brothers you and I, and it's perfectly fine if you turn out to be better-looking, faster, stronger, richer, bigger-penised, and generally more of a magnificent example of the species than I am. Good luck to you. It doesn't mean I don't have my own gifts to offer, however. Far from it. Indeed, may these gifts I humbly offer herewith in handbook form serve ye well. And may your lovers evermore cry out in joy.

Shout going out to all the gay men

If, for whatever reason, you got previously tripped up in all this barefoot doctor malarkey and thus presently find yourself flicking through these pages, I'd like you to know I think willies are great and that I include you when I write, trusting that with only the slightest use of imagination, you'll be able to adapt these techniques to suit yourself and derive as much benefit/entertainment as the heteros.

Shout going out to all the lesbians

I envy you sometimes. Much of my fundamental sexual inspiration and understanding of the female has come from hanging out with you over the years, watching you dance, kiss, and fondle one another. I hope you and all my dyke friends (especially Vivian) have fun with this material and find it easy to adapt and make use of the Yin and Yang of it all.

Shout going out to all the pervs, s 'n' m freaks, auto-eroticists, fetishists, and other assorted deviant adventurers

Though personally a sucker for absolute freedom of movement and freedom from pain for all parties involved in my "lovemaking" activities, I have extensively explored the above regions in deep and candid conversation with practitioners and by attending various parties and "orgies" around the planet, for both my personal and professional mind-expansion programs. And I think I've got a handle on what you're up to, more of which you'll find later in the book. It is my hope that the information presented will offer you new insights to help refine your pleasure and the possibility of alternative ways to express your love/need for love. It is also my hope that I haven't just offended you (rubber rules OK?).

Shout going out to all the old bastards
(and dears)

What are you doing looking at this, you naughty thing? Forgive me, young whippersnapper that I am, I still display the arrogance of (advanced) youth, but am, however, genuinely concerned about the sexual challenges facing us as we grow into our dotages.

I'm concerned both on a professional level, dotage-sex issues comprising a sizable chunk of my healing workload, and on a personal level, knowing full well that the years are racing by and it won't be more than the flicker of an eye before I myself am similarly challenged.

There are many fine snippets of useful information on offer herein intended to enhance dotage sex. After all, the great masters/mistresses of this art were traditionally in their nineties, at least.

And if there're any first-timers out there tonight . . .

Welcome to the minefield. If you think it's weird the first time, just wait. It's my sincere wish that this material encourages you to enjoy a lifetime of warm, caring, loving, erotically charged, scintillatingly stupendous sex, and that you may do so without guilt, shame, confusion, loss of personal integrity, or too much dishonesty, in health and pleasure for the next hundred years (or more).

What *is* a modern lover?

Anyone who's still got a pulse of some sort running through his/her sexual organs, who isn't sworn to a lifetime's celibacy, who happens to have seen through the trance of the fairy-tale 1950s Hollywood musical romance scenario, the matching polo shirts, jeans, and deck-shoes idyll of the nuclear family, the everything'll be fine once I'm married with kids delusion, and any other stereotyped walking off into sunsets happily ever after myths you may care to mention (and don't call me cynical, you know I'm speaking the truth), and who realizes that we're all engaged in a gargantuan sociological experiment, the outcome of which is wildly unpredictable at this time.

As you know, in the Western world, girls are beginning to outflank boys in the workplace and, more important, at school and college. They also now engage in the hitherto exclusively manly arts of boxing, wrestling, body-building, and gladiatorial contests of speed and strength. And technological sophistication makes it much easier to hunt the food, to haul the water and firewood, and to defend the realm (shucks, *anyone* can do it these days).

This obviously strips the boys of some of their former cachet and privileges and in short reduces their capacity for negotiating control in their relationships with women.

Other than for producing sperm, men are becoming a luxury rather than a necessity.

This has led to an intriguing situation.

The tenets of courtly love, which survived right through to the second half of the twentieth century, fueled to their absurd crescendo by the high-camp songwriting of such luminaries as the charmingly adroit Cole Porter, and based on the assumption that it was a man's world, had it that women were mere objects of men's desire (not fully fledged people in their own right). Beautiful women therefore became valued as great treasures, to be won (or paid for) at great price. Along with this female deification process went the mistaken belief that women didn't want sex (it was simply too rude), only men did. Though considering the ill-informed, sexually uncultivated natures of most of the male klutzes around at the time, this was probably true.

Nice girls just didn't do it. So other than spending time around un-nice girls, the only way to score big-time was to marry someone. Drastic measures indeed. But they held it (the marriage scenario) down in the main part, those brave suburban warriors. That is, until the 1960s socio-sexual revolution blew the lid off that particular Pandora's condom box of bourgeois, stiff-lipped hypocrisy.

Free love blossomed into full-blown promiscuity, degenerated into drug-augmented decadence, and led to a proliferation of the three H's (herpes, hepatitis B/C/D, and HIV) as well as the births of many people with names like Tarquin and Jemma.

Then came the reactionary backlash. People, and I'm talking twenty-five and younger, began feigning the adoption of a quasi-Victorian, pre-1960s set of morals. Promiscuity and decadence were a thing of the past, relegated to the politely twee environs of the monthly rubber club or swingers' night at your local disco. "Back to basic," i.e, back to potential hypocrisy, and a return to traditional family values, i.e, a return to love affairs on the sly, became the order of the day in the early 1990s.

However, by the late nineties, with premillennial syndrome raging, girls openly admitting how much they wanted sex, condoms readily available, and the drug cocktails rendering HIV more user-friendly, people were both "doin' it" and not doing it more than ever, and all at once, in every which way—neo-Victorian repressive, neo-1960s, swinging, bisexually, rubberizing, bondaging, discreetly, indiscreetly, discriminately, indiscriminately, lasciviously, demurely, cyber-spatially, not-until-we're-married stylee, let's just fuck now stylee—any and every way and nonway you can possibly imagine.

And the upshot is that everyone's a bit confused (sometimes). And no one's got the answer. The boys don't know where they stand. The girls don't know where they stand. Whichever way we're trying it, we acknowledge that the old ways are unsatisfactory. Marriage is no longer the original cornerstone of society. And try as we might, we can't yet find anything better with which to replace it (as a cornerstone, that is).

We finally admit that we're feeling our way in the dark here, you and I. And that's exciting.

Anyone who knows that excitement and is happy to be part of the grand experiment, whether singled or coupled, is a modern lover. Technically it should be post-postmodern lover, but that would have made an ungainly title for a handbook, don't you think, so I settled on modern.

Needless to say, it has nothing to do with the clothes you wear, music you dance/listen to, or clubs/bars/restaurants you frequent. We're all in this together, no matter how stylish you are.

But the point I was making was that with this development the gender roles have reversed somewhat, and now it's the boys who are the objects of desire. It's the boys who act all pristine and pure. And it's the girls seducing them, wondering if *they* might score tonight.

And that's fine too (I enjoy it anyway), as long as the boys don't let it turn them into bimbos.

So there's my justification, as if one were needed, for the use of "modern" in the title. My *reason* for using it, however, is simply that it has a fine ring—Modern Lovers, I mean.

The story of "O"

To avoid clumsy repetition of such dull and lusterless titles as lover, partner, playmate, etc., to designate the other person(s) you're trying this stuff out on, the other person will, from here on in, be known simply as "O," but without the quotation marks, as in O.

Use of the vernacular

You may have gathered that I find it cumbersome to write any differently from the way I speak in real-time/life. When discussing matters sexual, just like you (unless you're a real stiffy), I often use terms such as dick, cock, willy, pussy, fuck, going down, coming/come, French-kissing, soixante-neuf (69), and even cunt (in the right circumstances).

For the sake of decorum and good manners, however, I shall attempt to eschew the use of the vernacular and to use the original Latin terms wherever possible, unless I find it interrupts my flow, in which case, please be prepared for a few little shockers.

After all, these are only words we're playing with, and the very fact that we have designated these affectionate descriptions of our own body parts and sexual activities as taboo, only to be used as insults or "dirty" pillow talk, is indicative of the deep stream of sexual sickness running through our society.

Conversely, I'm not going to use the (revealing) expression "making love" instead of "fucking," just to prove I'm a nice guy (unless I *want* to).

My own personal motivations for presenting this material
(in case you want to know)

first motivation I'm a compulsive author and as such you've got to write about *something*.

second motivation Wilhelm Reich, the late, great, seminal psychophysical therapist, direct student of both Sigmund Freud and Carl Jung, who died in a U.S. prison, where he was incarcerated for being a subversive, wrote a seminal treatise, "Function of the Orgasm," which in a nutshell stated that the ability to enjoy a full, unfettered, no-holds-barred orgasm was a true barometer of both your psycho-emotional and physical health. The degree to which you can't let go and come fully is the degree to which your neuroses have a hold on you, my friend.

In my (extensive) work as a healer over the past twenty-one

years, I have found Reich right. It is quite evident that when someone's in a state of balance and health, energy flowing freely in the meridians, all seven chakras humming merrily away, they have big, thundering orgasms. But when their energy flow is impeded by tension or disease, neurosis or psychosis, they can't come properly, and if they do they feel bad about it right afterward.

In a way, you could say that included in my mission to spread healing, self-acceptance, relaxation, and inner/outer peace is embedded a submission to get the whole world coming like troopers.

third motivation The issue of interpersonal, intimate relationships between people, especially where sex has been, is, or will be involved, is one of the most interesting topics of discussion I know (how about you?), and I feel this handbook provides the perfect forum/milieu to air a few thoughts/ideas, having been privy to the secrets of tens of thousands of patients as well as to those of my own friends and lovers. None of which I would dream of divulging, naturally, but which altogether have given me a phat chunk of fuel to fire up the odd observation or two.

fourth motivation By sharing what does amount, without wishing to brag, to a vast storehouse of experience and knowledge on the subject of sexual love, I am freeing up some space on my personal hard disk, which I suspect will then propel me into a new realm of sexual love altogether. I have no idea what that might be, but I'm up for it—I'm a sucker for change.

fifth motivation It provides me with a vehicle for perpetrating a bit of mild controversy (I hope), which appeals to my inner cultural terrorist.

sixth motivation It could easily sell millions.

('Nuff motivations?)

How to take optimum advantage of the text

Read it (obviously). Assimilate it. Picture it, smell it, feel it. (This part's important, because you can't read it as you practice the techniques. Well you might be able to, but it's not strictly recommended, even if you read out loud in a very sexy voice to each other, as this generally leads to fits of pealing giggles and subsequent likely loss of blood from a hitherto engorged penis.)

Once you've read cover to cover, take bits at random, whether new perspectives or new moves, and try them the next time you have sex with O.

Obviously, the ideal would be for O to be doing likewise simultaneously. (Well, actually it would be if you, O, and everyone else were taught this stuff as kids at school—and this was the official textbook.)

Wayward Taoist philosophical premises and morals
(as if)

Modern Wayward Taoism is identical to original Taoism before it became known as such, when following the natural way of things (Tao) was the only thing for a natural person to do. Before artifice crept into the mix and life became one big Confucianist charade, people knew no other way to be. Subsequent to that golden era, as society grew more complex and self-conscious, people who followed the natural way became rarer and hence more remarkable, and as with all phenomena they needed a name, otherwise how could people bitch about them.

Now, I don't know how, but they called it "Tao," hence "Taoism," but true "Taoists" worth their cinnabar would be too absorbed in the "is" to be interested in "isms," and would wholeheartedly eschew the use of the title. Tao is free flowing; after all it comprises, among everything else, the entire known and unknown universe, so it has to remain pretty flexible. [See *The Tao*, p. 24.] Isms are traps, for as soon as you define something you tend to kill its essence.

However, as is the way with these things (if you'll excuse the pun), what with people loving to organize themselves into clubs/institutions/tribes, etc., in pre-Communist China, Taoism had actually degenerated into an intricate quasi-religious movement, complete with churches, liturgy, and its own papal figure.

Fortunately, the Taoist blueprint is elegantly contained and carried in various "structures" or forms which have survived more or less intact for thousands of years, even making a successful transition from the eastern to the western hemisphere without becoming too polluted (so far). In fact, some of these forms have become hugely popular, even fashionable in some quarters, and if packaged effectively constitute a highly salable "commodity." Some of the Taoist forms you may be familiar with are acupuncture, tai chi, and feng shui.

All the Taoist forms, however, including the magic, the meditations, the medicine, the martial arts, the sexology, originate from before the time Taoism got lost up its own ass, and are therefore pure carriers of the blueprint. And that's fine as long as you don't spend too much time defining it and institutionalizing it, otherwise you may kill it.

So, in response to the growing problem of Taoists around the globe, Wayward Taoism grew up of itself in North London, surfacing in the early 1990s, specifically at the Highgate Egg. The beautiful thing about Wayward Taoists (literally, wards of the way) is that most of them are so involved in it (the Tao), they don't even realize they're Wayward Taoists. They are the urban warriors and heroes/heroines who are experimenting with a new way, followers of the nu-skool of philosophy. Their numbers are legion. You're probably one yourself.

Their philosophy is do what you feel like. Be who you are. Not who you think you should be.

Their morals are treat yourself lovingly and treat others as you treat yourself.

Always.

Sex as a spiritual path

Sex is the most potent (voluntary) tangible expression of primal energy available for humankind to experience.

Violence is potent too, but as it only destroys, it is not as potent as sex.

Sex is creative—*and* it can destroy you. So it has both aspects, unlike violence. That's why sex beats violence every time.

When the Tao got pregnant and gave birth to the everything, it probably started with an urge not dissimilar to your own sexual urge when you want a little action.

What's inferred here is that the sexual urge is one with the original creative urge of existence itself. Think about it. It's how you make new people. Do you know any magic tricks better than that? (Not even David Blaine does.)

Sex is spiritual.

But as with any practice, it's all in how you enter the temple.

If you enter the temple and spit on the floor, you'll get a different hit from walking in filled with expectant awe.

The original Taoists knew this and cultivated a path which would enable the practitioner to enter the sexual temple in the appropriate way to elicit the desired outcome, which for them was total out-of-body, out-of-mind union at the highest level of consciousness with the Undifferentiated Absolute (Tao)—tripped-out bliss, in other words.

The original Taoists knew that if you entered the temple with the appropriate awareness, you could, through the shared experience of sexual love, refine your energy and consciousness to such a high degree that not only would you become enlightened through it, you'd become immortal to boot.

I'm sure you've heard about Tantric Sex—it's been getting good press lately—well, that's the Hindu/Buddhist version. It's more ritualistic and externally dramatic than its older Taoist sister, but essentially leads you to a similar state of sexual nirvana. [See *Sexual nirvana*, p. 67.]

Anyhow, it's the Taoist model that was miraculously passed down to this particular barefoot doctor (proving the Tao has a keenly developed sense of humor), and which I proudly pass on to you now. A Taoist, especially a Wayward one, never runs away from powerful urges through self-denial, renunciation, or any form of self-repression.

Instead, he/she goes with the urge and sublimates/transforms it through various feats of psychophysical inner alchemy (viz., what's on offer in this and previous handbooks) into a refined mix of energy, consciousness, and spirit.

Rather than deny the sexual urge (or any other primal urge), the Taoist uses it for enlightenment fuel. (Likewise, rather than deny the violent urge, the Taoist sublimates it by practicing tai chi and so on, i.e., he/she uses it for enlightenment fuel also.)

So rather than deny the fact that you want to wander down that slippery old sex path, walk freely but with awareness and you'll become enlightened too. (Please note, enlightenment through sex doesn't preclude confusion, heartbreak, and getting generally fucked up from time to time.)

(Please also note that, except in extreme cases, sex was never intended as the only spiritual path and is best blended and balanced with other spiritual paths, such as that of making a living, otherwise you'll just end up fucking and/or starving yourself half to death.)

The Tao

(The "T" of Tao is pronounced softly so it sounds almost like a "d," as in "Dow" Jones.)

Imagine before the universe began, there was Absolute Nothing(ness). Imagine Absolute Nothing developed a sexual urge, at first just a little tingle down below. But as no-time went by, this tingle began to grow, as these things do, until it became a definite rumble that was eventually so powerful that the whole of Absolute Nothing began to rattle and hum. What had started as an innocent trickle now became an irrepressible, irreversible tidal flood, shuddering to an overwhelming, irrevocable climax with only one way to go. Out. But as there was no out, because there was no in, and as there was absolutely no birth control then, Absolute Nothing impregnated itself and the universe was born nine months later. Big Bang, my ass (actually, don't).

(That's not the Tao. That's just a story.)

The Tao is too great/minuscule to even conceptualize one holographic cubic centimeter of it, let alone describe it. It can, however, be discerned hidden in the doings of your life when you follow/allow the natural way in all circumstances (especially sex), instead of trying to act/not act like you think you should/n't.

Hence the Tao is usually translated as "way." In Japanese it's pronounced "do" (doe) as in Aikido (the way of channeling ki or chi). Or Fido, my friend Suzuki's dog, for example.

The universe is consciousness made manifest

Otherwise how does the grass always know how to grow just so? Consciousness is everywhere, in the smallest atom of this book, in your hand as you hold this book, in your brain as you read it, in your friend's brain when you tell him/her about it, in the toilet paper you use if you're reading this in the bathroom, in the design of the toilet bowl, and in the words of William Shakespeare, Franklin D. Roosevelt, and Tom Robbins (for example).

Everything you see around you, every city, every planet, every Q-Tip you use to clean your ear holes, every sound you hear, every drill on every road, every (goddamn) car alarm outside your window, every smell your noble nose detects, every sensation everyone feels ever, started with a simple thought—consciousness made manifest.

This consciousness is ubiquitous, and it's what you're playing with when you have sex. The bodies are just there to give the experience a time and space fix/reference point in order for it to be made manifest. You can fairly accurately substitute "consciousness" for "Tao."

Yin and Yang

But the Tao was smart. (You've got to be when you take on a job like that.)

It observed that as soon as it brought forth an idea from the Absolute Nothing, in order to make it manifest in the visible universe, a polarity would be instantly generated. Say, for example, it wanted to bring forth into being a Swiss casserole dish. Once manifest, you'd have a Swiss casserole dish and, of course, its opposite, no Swiss casserole dish.

Just to be sure, the Tao tried it out with other phenomena, other values. It tried hot and discovered cold. It tried doing clever spinning and orbiting tricks with planets and suns to create the effect of daylight and discovered night. It also discovered, quite quickly in fact, that one pole of the polarity, once it had reached the zenith of its beingness, would automatically start to transform into the opposite pole.

Hence, the Swiss casserole dish, once it had reached the zenith of its dishness, finding itself on sale for thirty thousand Swiss francs in an antique shop in the old part of Geneva, for instance, was in fact already crumbling from within. Daylight, as it reached its noontime zenith, already contained the seeds of darkness and the time of day when it (the Tao) could, for a while, forget about all this creation shit and go to the nearest bar and get drunk.

The Tao noticed all this. It saw it everywhere, but was most interested to see it being acted out by people having sex together. It noticed the active penis thrust into the passive vagina get sucked in actively and pull away passively. It noticed that at various times during the session, the man would be active and the female passive, then they'd switch around.

From where the Tao was watching it looked like a fine conundrum, but it would have been rude to have got too close, so it sat back and took a deep breath. A name was needed for this dynamic, as it was obvious it was running throughout existence; a name that would sound like what it described (onomatopoeic). The Tao tried out a few contenders—Bill and Ben, Jack and Jill—and finally settled on Yin and Yang, came up with a logo/motif similar to two fish performing soixante-neuf, and it turned out to be a big hit.

Yin is generally used to describe the shadow, Yang the light. Yin is the receptive, Yang the active. Yin is the structure of a situation, Yang the force that animates it. Yin is the female, Yang the male.

These, however, are relative terms. A man has/uses Yin (female energy) as much as a woman has/uses Yang.

Hot is Yang. Cold is Yin. The sun is therefore Yang. A small candle flame is also hot, but compared to the sun is relatively cold, and is therefore Yin.

It is also true that Yin cannot exist without Yang. If there was no non-Swiss casserole dishness, the entire known universe would be one huge Swiss casserole dish. (It probably is, in fact.)

I mention this not just as sweet nothings whispered in your ear before we get down to business. It is important to appreciate the Yin and Yang of sex, as these terms will be used every now and then, often at crucial moments during the upcoming text.

Chi

Chi translates as "life force."

Chi is love in action. It's invisible. It moves through the air with the greatest of ease, like those magnificent men on their fly-ing trapeze.

Without it nothing would happen. Anywhere. Ever. At all.

When you love someone, what carries the feeling of love from you to them, so they can feel it, is chi. When you think of some-one you love, chi carries your thought to them. That's why they phone you out of the blue like that.

When the penis thrusts deeper and moans escape, it's chi in the pleasure that brings the pleasure home. Chi is the connective agent that travels everywhere throughout the universe all at once on behalf of its boss, Big Tao. Chi is consciousness's envelope.

Chi is flowing throughout your own body, even as you read this. It travels through channels termed meridians (by the French Jesuit missionaries who first imported Taoist knowledge to Europe). Acupuncture/acupressure (shiatsu) works by stimulating the flow of chi in your meridians. That's common knowledge these days. What isn't so common is the knowledge that chi goes wherever your thoughts go and will be as powerful as your mental focus. (That's how magic works.)

Imagine being able to send your chi/love up O's spine in a thrilling shock of pleasure and have O send it back twice as strong, just by thinking it.

That's the gist of the "drug" herein on offer [See *Whooshing the Chi*, p. 199.]

Balance

Obviously, balance is essential in everything you do, particularly in sex.

Over time you train yourself to be sensitive to the dynamic bal-ance of love and desire, holding and releasing, starting and stopping, foreplay and fucking, stroking and licking, kissing and sucking, pushing and pulling, hardness and softness, activity and passivity, giving and receiving, tension and relaxation, thrusting hard and merely wiggling about—Yin and Yang.

By sensitizing yourself to dynamic balance you automatically allow balance to establish itself, of itself. You don't have to do anything about it. Simply be aware. Allow balance to be and balance will balance itself out.

Obvious stuff indeed, but an awareness of balance, or at least the possibility of it, is crucial to developing an understanding of the Taoist love and sex scenario.

Love

I fear (which is the opposite of love, as you know) we cannot proceed further without some mention of the L word.

What is love?

You tell me.

My telling you what love is, is not only preposterous, it's downright arrogant.

If you don't know what love is, for you, you need help, buddy, help which I can't give you through words alone.

However, you could say that love is being open to someone. Simple as that. Being open, the chi can travel where and how it will between you.

You could say love is only wishing warmth, joy, and freedom to whoever it is you're loving.

You could say love is wishing no harm or limitation for whoever it is you're loving.

You could say love is what happens when you look O, or anyone for that matter, in the eyes and say, "I love you" (as you do).

You could say love comes from an open heart.

You could say God is love.

You could say a whole lot of things, but it'd be better to get hold of someone you love and give 'em a good squeeze.

Sexual love

Sexual love is what happens/passes between you when you have sex with O and you feel completely open to each other, without negative judgments about body shapes, smells, hairstyles, movement styles, vocal sounds, personality quirks, boudoir decor, etc.

On the contrary, you find yourself loving and/or liking the physicality of O as much as your own, and feel happy to be sharing yourself thus.

Sexual love happens when your loins, heart, and brain are wide open and receptive/generous in the presence of O while engaged in sexual activity. [See *The Three Tan Tiens*, p. 46.]

Recreational sex vs. procreational sex

Sex is obviously recreational. It's so enjoyable. Which is why people do it and think about it so often. You have the chance to re-create yourself every time you do it. What else could it be but recreational?

Procreational.

Babies are not just for Xmas, as any child/parent will tell you. Birth control is an essential factor to weigh in when considering engaging in sex with O.

But just because sex *can* create new people, it doesn't *have* to. There's nothing wrong and everything right about having sex just to engender mutual pleasure, especially if that practice can lead to enlightenment.

When practiced in the Taoist way, unless expressly wanting an actual pregnancy, sex is used to create new people out of you and O. Each orgasm is a rebirth.

This is just to say that there's nothing self-indulgent about refining your sex. If every squirt and shudder led to babies we'd all be falling into the sea by now.

Beauty

It seems rude to continue without talking of beauty.

One way or another, it's beauty we are worshiping when we truly share sexual love with O.

Beauty is only skin-deep. Well, cosmetic beauty is, but you should also take bone structure and connective tissue into account.

Beauty is in the eye of the beholder. So if there's no one beholding your beauty, does that mean you're not beautiful at that moment?

Beauty can be symmetrical. Beauty can be twisted. Beauty can even be ugly and ugly beautiful.

All things bright and beautiful are that way because beauty is an archetypal, a priori quality. It exists before we do. All that happens then is that with each successive generation that comes through the shoot, beauty is expressed through them anew. Beauty keeps reinventing itself as each successive generation passes. And though trends may change, beauty as a quality remains the same: beautiful.

When your soul is beautiful, i.e., mostly free of evil intention, beauty will shine through your eyes and animate your features. It will shimmy down the lines in your face and lend you an air of character. It will infuse your pheromones as they waft across a crowded room and it will add discreet harmonics to the timbre of your voice.

Beauty is a matter of taste. Taste the beauty in everyone. Especially everyone you sleep with. Watch them from close up as they moan and writhe in sexual ecstasy. That's beautiful.

But don't just celebrate O's beauty, celebrate your own too. If you have a problem channeling beauty (to your exterior), repeat the following affirmation endlessly until it becomes a pattern on the wallpaper of your mind: "I am beeeeyyooooootiful!"

All girls and boys are spiritual sisters and brothers, hence sex is incest on a grand scale

Realizing this makes sex both more compassionate and more naughty/exciting. It reduces your tendency to regard O as object rather than other.

All beings, at their roots, are one, hence sex is just the Tao jerking off

Realizing this takes the strain off your local, personal sexual melodramas. It takes the edge off your feelings of guilt and shame when you've fucked someone you shouldn't have. You were just doing it for the Tao. So next time you hear a big, phat voice, like rolling thunder calling from the clouds, asking you to pass the tissues, you'll know who it is.

Sex and connecting with the mystery of creation

Sex is one of the most direct ways of connecting to the common life force and thereby entering the mystery of creation. That's why people are so constantly drawn there, whether they know it or not.

When you share sexual love you are connecting with each other, that's obvious. What you are also doing is, together, connecting to the source of life itself—the Tao.

If you actually take time to notice that, it transforms your shared sexual experience, instantly taking it down to a much deeper level. If, in addition, you refine your awareness of the life force plugged into and released during sex, you can utilize it to increase the excitement, light up your brain, and ultimately induce an orgasm of such universal proportions that when you come, the entire solar system shudders with you, rolls over, and takes a nap. You enter the timeless state (beyond limited concepts of linear time) of sexual nirvana.

It is extremely good for your health, spiritually, energically, emotionally, and physically, to do this, and it is even claimed by some to reduce facial wrinkles.

Of course it works best, i.e., creates synergy, when both you and O are consciously sharing this awareness, but the true magic of this stuff is that it works fine if just one of you does it—both you and O will get the big bang. In other words, only one of you needs to be practicing the tricks set out in the upcoming text for both of you to get the payoff.

You're free to do
whatever you choose

According to the Wayward Taoist scheme of things, you are perfectly at liberty to enjoy sex with whomever you choose, as long as
they are willing, of sound mind, and legally within limits, whenever and however you (both) like, as long as you do it with love
(and respect).

If this involves lying and/or breaking agreements with other
lovers, there will eventually be consequences, not as divine punishment (only you can punish yourself), but as agents of change
and transformation to help you grow. [See *Lying/denying*, p. 100,
and *All is fair in love and war*, p. 101.]

Not necessarily good,
not necessarily bad

This is a basic tenet of Wayward Taoism. What looks good today
can look like shit tomorrow, and vice versa.

You win the jackpot. Your friends say, "Congratulations." You
say, "Not necessarily good." They think you're being blasé. Soon
after, through restlessness and ennui, you become a raging alco-
holic. Your friends say, "That's awful." You say, "Not necessarily
bad." Your friends think you're stupid. In the rehab center, you
meet a healer (maybe a barefoot doctor) who shows you how to tap
the spiritual stream, your life is transformed, and soon you become
a famous guru. Your friends marvel and say, "Well done, who would
have thought it." You say, "Not necessarily good." They think
you're just making spiritual wisecracks because you're so enlightened. Two months later, the Chinese take over and all gurus are

rounded up and forced at gunpoint to do pirouettes in the sunset on Venice Beach. ('Nuff said?)

In other words, desist immediately from judging yourself, others, and/or situations you encounter as either good or bad. You cannot possibly enjoy a huge enough perspective upon which to draw up your list of criteria and hence be able to form a valid opinion. Only the Tao can do that. And even the Tao doesn't judge because the Tao's enlightened and it knows that all judgments are relative to time and place, i.e., subject to limited perspective.

Once you stop judging/limiting yourself, others, and/or situations, once you stop coming from your list of spurious, subjective criteria, you make space for yourself, others, and/or situations to develop magically/exponentially. This especially applies to the entire sexual love dance (seduction—sex—snoring).

The nonsense of morals

Because sex is the most potent primal force voluntarily accessible to humankind, the most potentially creative and destructive, every social grouping ever to have graced the ground with its footsteps has attempted to impose rules governing the sexual activities of its members. These rules vary wildly. In some cultures a woman has two or more husbands. In other cultures she is publicly beheaded for the same behavior. In some cultures a man has four wives, in others he's called a bastard.

Different cultures have different rules. Some, but not all, are written, while many are merely tacitly assumed and loosely known as moral codes. These moral codes are often unfathomable and tend to lead to severe confusion. (Especially when spoken about.)

The only constant, unchanging factor, the only common

denominator in all this, is that *everybody* transgresses their moral code (to some extent at one time or another).

Hypocrisy consists of pretending that isn't so for you.

So what we have is everybody, at some time or other, doing whatever they can get away with, because they feel like it, completely regardless of any moral code, while simultaneously maintaining a pretense of abiding by the rules. It's called acting.

(I naturally make allowances for this generalization to be proven invalid. I do, however, base my view not only on personal experience but also on the—approximately—sixty-four thousand cases I've treated over the past twenty-one years, wherein I've been privy to the secrets of nearly that many people, and though I wouldn't for a minute divulge those secrets, I feel perfectly at liberty to use the information to fuel my observations. And I can tell you, nobody's totally clean, my friend.)

Morals are like cosmetics. They merely mask the ravages beneath the surface. So while all the ravaging's going on, in friends' borrowed apartments on a working afternoon, for example, we all agree, mostly, to uphold this flimsy yet gooey veneer.

The sexual urge is too strong for most mere mortals to contain for long. It was always intended that way to ensure our species' survival. Sooner or later it has to burst free, and when it does, morals dissolve into the ether from whence they came.

Morals often make no true sense, but they do provide an interesting theatrical device, without which life might become a bit dull. Imagine *Safe Liaisons*. It doesn't exactly fire the imagination in the same way.

The only valid moral a Wayward Taoist is concerned with is: treat yourself with absolute love, kindness, and respect, treat others the way you treat yourself, and don't ever deviate far from that.

All the rest, as far as this Wayward Taoist can tell, doesn't bear close scrutiny, i.e., it is a pile of shit.

Relationships, the illusion of

Show me your relationship. Where is it? I see you. I see O. I see you relating to each other. But I don't see a relationship. You talk about this relationship as if it's the third party in a triangle. You, O, and the relationship. But where is it?

Surely you've noticed by now that the relationship is nothing more than a construct of your mind. And O's got one too, which is actually and obviously different from yours. And yet there you both are, in the *same* relationship. It would be more accurate to say there are four of you: you, O, your concept of the relationship, and O's concept of the relationship. That's four of you in the same bed. No wonder you get in such a pickle sometimes trying to get it all to harmonize.

There is in reality no such thing as a relationship. There is merely you, spending time, more or less regularly and/or frequently, relating with O. That's it. The rest is just your expectations, fantasies, and fears.

Knowing this helps you feel much freer, whatever your circumstances.

So stop looking for a relationship, the right relationship, the wrong relationship; stop looking to change your relationship or leave your relationship. Because relationships don't exist. You're wasting your time. Just shut up and play the record.

In other words, revel in the mystery of your one true relationship, i.e., the relationship you have with yourself, your higher self, or the Tao (if you want to get romantic about it), and when the Big Mystery throws an O in your path (who is similarly engaged in a relationship with O's self/higher self/Tao), do all you can to support him/her in that relationship and not get in the way. Support O with love. Support O with respect. Support O without expectation of reward. And value each and every moment of every encounter/relating session with O, whether it's the first encounter or the nine thousandth, as if it's a precious gift from the Tao (which it is), no matter how hard that may be sometimes.

Relating is an active phenomenon and hence fresh every time. Relationships are just bullshit in your mind.

Being/feeling sexy

What's not sexy, except in the eyes of a complete deviant, is having a belly full of wind and needing to fart, being constipated, needing to pee badly, having bad breath, soiled underwear, dandruff, smelling generally foul, spitting on the floor indiscriminately, vomiting, having visible boogers in your nose or snot streaming out, foaming at the mouth, suffering from a herpes attack on either the mouth or genitals, or having smelly feet.

These and other examples of what is not sexy (to most of us) notwithstanding, being sexy, i.e., being perceived by others as being sexy, arises purely from feeling sexy. It may just be an old wives' tale that the sexiest women are the ones who masturbate most, but I've personally always found it to be the case.

The more comfortable you are with your own sexuality, the more sexy you'll feel and the more sexy you'll be.

Obviously, sexy is different for different people (at different times). But generally the way to increase your sexiness is to repeat as often as you can, and I can't repeat this often enough, "I feel sexy." Say this to yourself over and over until you feel a subtle tingle somewhere between your upper thighs, or until you just feel sexy. Repeat this procedure on a regular basis for the next eighteen days or so. This is crucial, as feeling sexy is essential to partaking in truly satisfying sex.

Above all, be confident in your sexiness.

Visualize an energy channel beginning in the sole of each foot, running up the inside of both legs, meeting at the perineum (between your legs) and extending to the tip of the penis/uterus. Now visualize another channel running from the tip of the penis/uterus back to the perineum, dividing into two, running along your inguinal canals (the

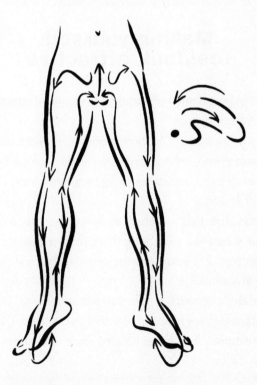

diagonal grooves which separate upper thighs from belly), and down the outside of both legs into the sole of each foot.

Breathe in and imagine/feel the breath entering through the soles, traveling up the inside of each leg into the perineum all the way to the tip of the penis/uterus.

Breathe out and imagine/feel the breath return to the perineum, separate into two streams along your inguinal canals, and travel down the outside of each leg to the soles of your feet.

Repeat this procedure nine times, slowly and deliberately saying to yourself, "I feel sexy," as the breath moves up, and "I am sexy," as the breath moves back down.

Repeat this every morning and night for ninety days and observe how people start responding differently to you.

Making yourself feel/look attractive

It's nothing to be ashamed of; sometimes you need external help in your quest for sexiness.

You may think it's sexy to sport greasy, messy hair, with sleep in the corners of your eyes and grime beneath your nails. You may think you look more attractive in egg-stained clothes. But most prospective Os won't.

Give yourself a fighting chance. Boost the economy. Go out and buy a new outfit or two. Something that makes you feel grand when you wear it. Pay some attention to your hairstyle (not just to your head) and nails.

Don't be shy of cosmetics. They're not shy of you. Don't be deluded into thinking it's unspiritual somehow to make the very best of your appearance. You came here to shine and shine you must.

It's your duty as a human. And if from time to time you need a few props to help the show along, then so be it. Use them well.

Feeling like you look good, especially when you undress for sex, is an immeasurable boost to your confidence, one less thing to fret about, and it allows you to relax so you can enjoy the main event more.

Whatever his/her destination, a modern lover always leaves home ready to get laid.

Vanity/self-consciousness

Never, however, allow vanity or self-consciousness to block your sexual flow of activity. Taking pride in your appearance is not the same as taking your appearance seriously. Your appearance is only that. It's not who you are. *You're* not even who you are. For who you really are is too big to fit in a (little) human form. All that shows is the tiniest fraction of who you are: your local self. To take this local self of yours seriously is like the World Trade Center taking one of its bricks seriously. Which isn't to say a brick shouldn't look as good as it can. By all means shine, but remember it's not you, your local self, who generates and provides the light. It's your great (universal) self who does that, i.e., the Tao. (Veiled clue to enlightenment.)

Hygiene

Shall I be polite here, or just tell it like it is?

Tell it like it is, Doc.

OK. There's nothing worse than going down on someone (male/female) whose genitals smell of various combinations of stale urine, rotting carp, Gouda cheese, this morning's bowel movement, and ammonia. It's horrible.

Be free-flowing, not just with your energy but with the soap/shower gel too. Be reckless with the toothpaste and irresponsible with the shampoo. Wash carefully, especially before, and eventually after sex. Go right inside all the secret places, wash everywhere/everything. Don't be shy of your own body. Merge with the soap/gel, be at one with the water.

Do not, however, take this as an invitation to fuel any compulsive-obsessive self-cleansing/purging patterns you may be prone to. Don't wash so much that you smell like a bottle of Pert Plus. Simply show yourself and others the personal respect you would expect them to show you.

Smells/scents

This is a touchy topic for most people. Everyone has their own angle on smell. The key is to find the right smell to augment your natural body odor rather than mask it.

Women in southern Spain traditionally rubbed a small amount of their own vaginal juices behind their ears and into their temples, mixed with delicate essence of jasmine, neroli, myrrh, ylang-ylang, or frangipani. They adopted this technique from the Moors, who inherited it originally from Taoist mistresses in ancient China, via the silk road.

Try it for yourself, gender permitting.

Wear scent sparingly to avoid O and others swooning unnecessarily. It can be unnerving to walk away from a tryst smelling like a perfumery.

Props/setting

Location and timing permitting, if you have the opportunity to do some set-building before commencing sexual proceedings, pay attention to clean sheets, subtle incense, ambient lighting with an emphasis on an absence of direct bright light shining in anyone's eyes, an easily accessible supply of sympathetic tunes ready in a nearby stereo, unless you can afford a troupe of sympathetic musicians, in which case they should be discreetly sequestered behind a screen, and a ready supply of condoms, if appropriate, under the pillow. [See *The vast importance of condoms*, p. 104.]

Obviously, this is at your discretion, but for Taoist sex, the employment of any other props—tools, toys, bondage/entrapment equipment, instruments of pain, rubber/leather costumes, French maids' outfits, fruit and vegetables, etc.—is normally eschewed, as the emphasis is on what goes on internally for both/all of you and not on external objects/fetishes. Not that there's anything wrong with all that shit, it's just that it becomes irrelevant and tends to create clutter.

Stop performing and start feeling

As you may have noticed, it's easy for sex to degenerate into a performance. You find yourself performing not just for O but for a greater (imaginary/internalized) audience.

Sometimes you may find yourself moaning/groaning because it seems appropriate, rather than because you can't help it. You may find yourself moving your body according to a script and doing things to O because you think it may be expected, rather than moving and doing spontaneously.

And if you're doing it, you can be sure O's doing it too, because nowhere do we provide such clear/precise mirrors for each other as when we're having sex.

But that's fine. Everyone does it from time to time, even if only momentarily.

It's just that when you're in performance mode, you're not in feeling mode. When you're not in feeling mode, you can't feel what's going on. You can see it, you can sense it through your skin, you can smell it, and you can hear it, but you can't *feel* it, because you're removed, you're in your head and not your body.

That's why, when you do it as a performance, you need O's feedback afterward, like needing the applause, because you weren't really there for the main event and are therefore left undernourished.

Drop the performance, however professional your delivery may be, and start feeling what's going on from the inside. Then you can feel where your body wants to go next, rather than trying to follow an imaginary script.

This doesn't, however, preclude the enactment of your fantasies in blow-by-blow detail, when appropriate. [See *The nature of pure sexual intelligence vs. fantasy*, p. 56.]

Enacting the eternal dance of Yin and Yang

Yin and Yang, the receptive and the creative, the nucleus and the electron, the egg and the sperm, the full and the empty, are the two primordial forces/aspects of Tao, which together provide the basis for physical existence.

Yin (equating to emptiness) and Yang (equating to fullness) are engaged in an eternal dance, which until existence draws itself to a close, will go on forever.

Yin takes, Yang gives. Yin is full now and Yang is empty. This means they have reversed roles. Yin then gives and Yang takes. This means they have reversed roles again. Yin becomes Yang and Yang becomes Yin and they keep doing this again and again (without ever suffering from ennui).

Sensitizing yourself to this dance is important. As humans we enact the dance of Yin and Yang here on earth. We can't help it, we're like puppets in this respect.

What we can help, however, is the elegance and grace with which we express the movement of Yin and Yang, both within us as individuals and between us when having sex with Os.

To find your own elegance and grace in the expression of the dance, you must first be aware of which phase you're in, so you can start to discern the given rhythm and follow it. For example, when you find yourself doing all the doing and O just lying there being done to, you are in the extreme Yang phase and O is in the extreme Yin. If this pattern is repeated regularly, your own Yin will be drained, and unless O engages with you in a couple of sessions of doing all the doing to you, you may find yourself going elsewhere to replenish your Yin.

It is important to remember, when attempting to decipher the above example, that Yin, though representing the female energy, does not automatically represent the woman. It can do, but it can also just as easily refer to the man. Same for Yang.

Yin represents the receptive or passive (and therefore the empty, as in standing by to receive). Yang represents the generating or active (and therefore the full, as in standing by to give). So when one man fucks another, the one getting fucked is mostly in the Yin phase, while the one fucking is in the Yang, even though both are male or Yang in relation to women.

More love

Love is the glue that holds reality together. Love provides the environment in which the dance is danced.

Love is not to be confused with sentimentality.

Love is not to be confused with being nice to each other.

Love is the willingness to be fully present, available, and open in a respectful, caring way, to the person and/or situation you currently find yourself dealing with. In the expression of sexual love, this openness and availability tend to extend to most/all entrances/exits of your physical person.

But to avoid getting entangled in the abstract, it is useful for our purposes here to acquaint yourself with the inner alchemical "mechanics" of your body. For it is through these that love is generated.

The Three Tan Tiens

According to the Taoist scheme (Wayward and Traditional), occupying the same so-called space of your physical person is an entity called your Immortal Spirit Body.

The Spirit Body is latent until activated. Or, more precisely, your awareness of your Spirit Body is latent until activated.

Once activated, however, your whole reality is instantly transformed and you take on both the inner landscape and mantle of a superhuman, with complete telepathic intelligence and absolute control over your chi.

When you're in this space while having sex, you transpose the experience of sexual love up a few quantum octaves, both for you and O, even if O doesn't have a clue what you're up to. If O's consciously doing it too, however, you create a synergy which bestows total empowerment on both of you simultaneously.

Sold?

Now, the way you activate Spirit Body awareness is by organizing your mind around, i.e., focusing on, what's known in the trade as your Three Tan Tiens.

The Three Tan Tiens are like three huge, mysterious psychic orbs which form the core supporting structure of your Spirit Body. In the "space" of your physical person, these orbs are "located" along the front of your spinal column.

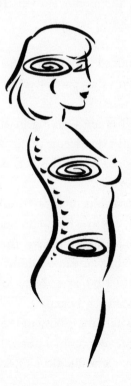

the lowermost tan tien is just below your navel and governs, among other things, your ability to generate and experience sexual desire, i.e., lust.

the middlemost tan tien is behind the center of your breastbone and governs, among other things, your ability to generate and experience passion, i.e., excitement, enthusiasm, and warmth.

the uppermost tan tien is bang in the middle of your brain, exactly where your pineal gland sits, and governs, among other things, your ability to generate and experience wishes/fantasies/pictures in your head, and moreover to discriminate between what you want and don't want to act out.

Tan Tien (pronounced something like "dunshiehn") means "heaven-field," implying that part of you is directly plugged into the great spiritual upstairs.

Ideally, the three TTs are working in absolute harmony with each other, exerting an even degree of governance over your lust, passion, and intelligence. When this occurs there is love, that is, you are in a state of love.

And the way you do this is simply to think about these three locations simultaneously (belly, chest, and head), with awareness of whatever physical sensation you have there, and to hold that thought as constantly as you can while having sex. By thinking about the three TTs (TTTs), your body relaxes and Spirit Body awareness is automatically activated.

Put another way, when chi is busy in the lowest TT, at the expense of the upper two, your animal lust will be strong, but it will be cold and brutal (deficient middle TT), without any discernible story line to follow (deficient upper TT). Rape results from extreme cases of this.

When both the lowermost and uppermost TTs are busy at the expense of the middle, your sex will be cold/clinical/brutal, i.e., without passion, but will follow an interesting story line. This engenders the sort of sex that is the enacting of pornographic fantasies.

When the lower and middle TTs are busy at the expense of the uppermost, your sex will be lusty and passionate, but without any intelligent awareness, and you'll probably forget everything that happened afterward. Excess alcohol intake is used to produce this amnesiac effect. This is like hot but slobby sex, the kind after which the guy usually rolls over and starts snoring.

When the upper two TTs are busy at the lowest TTs' expense, you won't be having sex anyway because erections/lubrication will be thin on the ground.

The balance of chi passing through the TTTs is constantly shifting, and the idea is to hold it steady and evenly distributed. Only one of you need maintain this awareness, as this will set up an energetic field which directly affects O. Obviously, if both you and O carry the awareness, synergy is created and the true magic can happen.

Also, by being sensitive to your own TT balance, you naturally become sensitive to O's TT balance, which is helpful when you're trying to fire things up, in that you know better where to send the fire.

Sharing consciousness

Whether you're sharing time with someone in a personal/intimate situation, family situation, business situation, sporting situation, martial arts situation, social situation, therapy situation, artistic/creative/musical situation, showbiz situation, or sexual-loving situation, what you are sharing during that time is consciousness.

Of all sharable situations, other than being born or dying, the sexual-loving situation is probably the most intense, intricately/delicately balanced and potentially enjoyable, with playing live music (at least for me) a close runner-up in the consciousness-sharing stakes.

When sexual love is firing up and animating every cell in your body, and your body is curling and writhing and squeezing and entwining itself with a similarly fired-up and animated O, and when the TTTs of both you and O (making six TTs altogether) are in full functioning mode, you're sharing consciousness at its most refined, spiritual level.

Sex is not about a dance of two or more bodies. Sex is a dance of minds/spirits, i.e., consciousness. The bodies are just there so you can both/all experience the proceedings on the physical plane. Call it gross if you will, but until you progress to angel form it's the best/highest level of interaction you're likely to encounter while still in possession of a physical form. (So make the most of it while you can.)

Eroticism

Cupid is cute, but Eros is fucking sexy. Eros is the god and hence provider of The Erotic Moment (TEM).

Eroticism is that which occurs during TEM.

Eroticism is not generated by the touching of skin on skin, nor upon the mixing and exchange of bodily secretions, but may include and indeed be the cause of these.

Eroticism is not generated at all, at least not by us. You can't contrive TEM. TEM just happens of itself in its own good time, at just the right time, when all prevailing conditions, including pheromone emission rates and wind speed/drag are juxtaposed in such perfect equipoise that Eros finds it impossible not to make an entrance.

Of course, your consciousness has to be available to notice the erotic presence (Eros) when it appears. Telltale signs are a shift in the tone of the lighting and colors around you, suddenly sharpened sensory perception, quickening pulse, a mild/medium/strong rise in adrenaline levels, most noticeable in the chest, slight acceleration of the breath, mild/imperceptible perspiration on the upper lip, possible stirrings amid the loins, and a little/not-so-little voice in your head, saying, "Wake up, something's happening here, girl/boy."

Always be sensitive to the erotic presence. Always be ready for TEM. TEM usually self-triggers when you make a move across a boundary. It can be an extra millisecond of a look held; the subtle crack in your voice as you tentatively but audaciously ask, "Do you want to . . . ?"; the sound of a whispered, "Yes," massaging the inside of your middle ear; as your fingertips fall softly, as if by accident, on the light downy hair on a forearm; in the moment I catch you starting to blush . . .

During the sexual dance, there will be moments that you (and it usually feels like both of you) feel the divine grace of erotic presence surround and engulf you. The etheric web that connects you to each other is clearly visible and appears charged with supraconsciousness.

Sometimes these erotic moments will last for a minute, sometimes for sixty-one minutes or more. When TEM comes, do not grab on to it. Be in a state of gratitude, i.e., receptive to grace, about it. Let it come. Let it go.

The purpose of Taoist sexual practice is not to engender The Erotic Moment. Its purpose is to engender rapid enlightenment-factor increase. But it is valid to say that it's likely you'll experience the erotic presence (Eros) more frequently, the more you practice Taoist sex.

Acting out vs. containment
to be or not to be, that is the question.
to do or not to do, that is the choice.

Eroticism is not necessarily to do with acting out a desire. It can be, but it is often more to do with containing the desire instead.

When faced with the choice of whether or not to act out a desire with someone you know you shouldn't, and you've entered that rarefied atmosphere of being temporarily beyond conscience about it, trust your body to respond appropriately and simply follow that response without getting in the way too much. Go with the moment, in other words, and trust your body to go only as far as it wants to. [See *Stopping when you want*, p. 134.]

Your body's truth is the only truth you can rely on. The rest is all idealism, which may or may not coincide with your real-time actions. But what your body does, where your body takes you, is where you actually go.

Maybe there is no choice. Maybe your choices are all predestined. Maybe it's all in the movement of the planets around the sun. Maybe the only choice is whether to relax or tense yourself while you experience the actions the desires in your body lead you to.

And when I say your body, I don't mean your dick or clitoris. I mean all TTTs working in harmony, saying, with one voice, from deep inside your bowels, "Do this/Do that," so unignorably that you find yourself engaged in activities which could profoundly alter the course of your life for a while.

You may well ask, is spiritual freedom found in acting out a desire or in containing it?

But what are you asking me for? I don't know. Is it?

The nature of desire

Desire is a powerful primordial force. It seems to arise out of nowhere and creep up on you from the inside. If you're not paying attention, it grabs hold of your mind and takes over. Now you are led by your desire like a bull with a ring through its nose. You are no longer free to enjoy your hitherto peaceful balanced view of your world/life. Instead you are slave to the whims of desire. And if the whim of your desire is to see him/her straightaway you'll drop everything else you're doing, no matter how important it was prior to that moment, and rush to his/her arms. You *know* that's true.

What you may not know is that the way to prevent this, when appropriate, and consequent acts of possible good-sense abandonment is immensely simple.

Mindfulness.

Be alert to desire as it initially arises. Do not under any circumstances deny its existence. To do so forces it into underground terrorist mode and lands you in all kinds of unnecessary trouble. Acknowledge desire without moral judgment.

Even if it's to fuck your best friend's mother/daughter/son/father/girlfriend/boyfriend or worse. Simply say, "Hello, Desire, and how are you today?" "Strong," comes the reply. "Well, I hearya," you respond, "but as you know, it might be impractical to

✦ **Barefoot Doctor's**

act you out today. I might have to contain and sublimate you for more mutually beneficial use."

"Mighty succinct and decent of you, as long as you're not just using all that highfalutin psychobabble to put me off," replies your now mildly paranoic desire.

After your initial negotiations with desire are complete, you can proceed to phase two of the operation: breathe (freely, deeply, and slowly).

Phase three is to say to your own higher self/spirit/personal Tao, "Take this desire and manifest it for me in the appropriate form for everyone involved to benefit and be life-enhanced thereby." Then let it go.

Phase four is to sit and watch what happens. (That's the fun bit.)

This four-stage Wayward Taoist desire management technique can, with practice, be performed in the mere twinkling of an eye.

So there you are, wondering whether to take your hand and lightly caress the side of O's face, or just keep it to yourself and remain politely platonic friends. Entirely unobserved, you complete phases one through four within one comfortable breath cycle. Suddenly, without warning, your left hand starts to lift, as if by its own accord, and floats slowly but deliberately through the gulf of air separating it from the side of O's face, where, upon landing, it gently strokes, with gossamer touch, that silken/shaven/bearded cheek. Without warning, O then gives you a hard slap on your own face and says, "Keep your hands off me, buddy, we're just friends. Remember?!" (You can't win 'em all.)

Try and control desire and it'll take control of you. Try not to control desire . . . and it'll take control of you.

Forget control altogether. (Except for lightly controlling your diaphragm as you perform each and every exhalation.) Instead, simply breathe and observe. Breathe and observe. Whether containing or acting out a desire. And remind yourself when caught in the viselike grip of a strong one, that a desire is only a desire, no matter for whom or for what. Keep breathing and eventually all desire will pass (so they say).

Ultimately all desire is the desire to go home (wherever/whatever that is for you). If you're stuck for somewhere to go, try your lowermost Tan Tien. This is where desire originates so it's a good place for it to go back to.

To experience the nature of desire as an abstract force, imagine you have a breathing aperture fitted directly into the center of your lower abdomen, just below your navel. As you inhale and exhale, feel the air stirring the force of desire in your lower TT. This may take up to twenty-nine breaths or more to accomplish.

The nature of passion

Broken dreams. Broken promises. That's usually where passion leads you. But that's no reason to run away from it. Better broken dreams than no dreams at all. And promises, as you know, are only made to be broken; there's no other reason to make them.

Your passion is too great to be confined within the limits of your dreams, and too wild to be trapped within the dubious moral context from which you draw the substance of your so-called promises. Even if the Tao itself tapped you on the shoulder and bade you promise to do, have, and be everything you want, every moment, for the rest of your life, and put it all on its tab, and you promised, you'd still break even on that one from time to time. So don't tell me about promises. No, what we want around here is passion.

For without passion, life would be too dull to mention. There'd be no real art to look at, no stirring tunes to hum, no love stories, not even any good sex . . . I mean, what the fuck would we do all day, what would be the point?

Passion is generated, governed, and physically experienced in the middle TT, located behind the center of your breastbone. Unbridled passion is potentially disruptive. It flambés your heart energy, which in turn flambés your mind and makes you nothing but a crazy fool to passion.

The best is to be giving full-flow to the generation and experience of passion, while at the same time bridling it by synchronizing its activity with activity in your lowermost TT, to give it physical expression, and with activity in your uppermost TT, to give it mental shape.

To touch and subsequently deepen the true nature of passion within you, imagine a breathing aperture fitted directly into the center of your chest. As you breathe in and out, feel as if the air thus entering and egressing is psychophysically stirring passion in your middle TT. This may require eighteen breaths or more.

The nature of pure sexual intelligence vs. fantasy

Desire stirs in your loins (lowest TT), fires up the passion in your heart/chest (middle TT), and the flames dart upward toward the center of your brain (upper TT), activating pure sexual intelligence/awareness. You are now "in" your Spirit Body and ready/primed for sharing sexual love.

If it should conveniently happen that O is similarly disposed/primed, you have the possibility of engaging in the sacred dance of Spirit Bodies that leads to sexual nirvana.

If, however, it should transpire that O is not similarly disposed, or even physically present, the situation therefore offering no actual possibility of imminent consummation, it is likely, unless you're already a dab hand at meditation, that the energy in your upper TT will seep forward into the frontal lobes of your forebrain and activate imaginary pictures/fantasies instead. [See *The question of masturbation*, p. 129.]

Pure sexual intelligence is only active when you are fully present in the moment and is that which enables your body to know exactly how to respond to another body, how to move just so.

Fantasy is only active when you are not fully present in the moment. The very nature of fantasy is that it takes your presence out of the moment into fantasyland.

There is nothing wrong about fantasizing. It's inevitable. Mostly, however, engaging in fantasy tends to lead to agitation.

There is nothing necessarily right about being fully present in the moment, either. It does, however, tend to lead you out of agitation, back into a state of calm.

The choice is yours (from moment to moment). You can have the present moment or you can have the fantasy. (It's your call.)

The trick is to allow and notice the fantasy as it arises, but then to breathe and allow it to subside, just like any other thought. It's following the fantasy that leads to delusion, agitation, and the self-polluting, thunderous crime against nature: masturbation, which, as you know, leads to epilepsy, St. Vitus' dance, mania, sensations of ants crawling down your spine, blindness, clammy hands, and eventually premature death (kidding).

Fantasies arise in a flash and often disappear again without trace, as when you notice a potential/real-life O in a coffee shop. And though you continue to sip daintily and even maintain the conversational pace with your friends, your mind is thinking, "God, how I'd like to squeeze that ass," and is picturing every detail with complete sensory enhancement. And all in half a twinkling of an eye. Sometimes, unless you're being particularly mindful in that instant, you won't even notice the fantasy go by.

Fantasies are essential. Spending time fantasizing about something/someone enables you to make a considered guess as to whether you'd like to invest the time/energy/money in making the object of your fantasy a manifest reality.

Even during the sexual dance itself fantasy plays an essential role in guiding your steps. While French-kissing O, you get a picture of yourself licking O's clitoris/glans, and a moment later you've shifted your physical orientation and now find yourself in a forest of pubic hair. It seemed fully spontaneous to the naked eye, but in reality you saw a picture/fantasy, then after a momentary delay, while you processed the picture and made a choice to act it out, you followed the picture with the actions of your body.

During the sexual dance, the key (as opposed to the trick) is to balance fantasy and pure sexual intelligence, oscillating between the two deftly, lightly, and swiftly enough to feel as if you're mostly centered in pure sexual intelligence. See the picture (forebrain-fantasy mode), but as soon as you follow it flip into pure sexual intelligence (mid-brain) mode so you can be fully present to experience/enjoy what transpires.

Honor your fantasies and fantasizing faculty as these give you the clues needed to take you to your next adventure/part of the adventure. But do not mistake them for manifest reality. Conversely, do not mistake manifest reality for fantasy just because you were too drunk/stoned/mashed to remember what you got up to last night and with whom, for that is often how unwanted pregnancies, sexually transmitted diseases (STDs), and weird people phoning who you wish wouldn't come about in your life.

The significance of smell

As important as the visual signals hitting the attraction receptors in your brain and sparking up your fantasizing faculties, are the subtle olfactory signals we send out. Everybody has a unique smell, more or less subtle, varying within certain parameters according to current state of health, time of month/year, generated by hormonal secretions, emitted through the pores of the skin, and carried in little spaceships called pheromones. Pheromones are minute information carriers which give the recipient nose the entire sexual blueprint of the sender. This information is retrieved and assimilated by the unconscious mind via the recipient nose's owner (or conscious mind if sensitivity-enhanced via regular meditational practice). Then, if your unconscious mind likes the smell and the smell likes your unconscious mind, and providing you've got an adequate line of chat and are not wearing funny shoes or anything else off-putting, you've probably got yourself a willing O for tonight.

On the other hand, you may also have had that disquieting experience of meeting someone to whom you were immensely visually, and even intellectually, attracted, but whom you found you had little or no physical desire for when push came to shove/love. This was because your pheromonal situations were somehow inequitable, i.e., you didn't like their smell.

And as you know, it's not always subtle, the smell I mean. Sometimes, the gross, consciously experienced smell of someone can put you off. But it can also attract you. Have you ever found the cheesy smell of a day's accumulated perspiration and toxin release between someone's toes strangely, secretly enticing? No? (Because I know a girl who could make men go crazy just by taking her sneakers off in public. Mind you, she was/is also awfully pretty, which might have tipped the balance in her favor somewhat.) [See *Hygiene*, p. 41.]

When wearing scent, choose one which will enhance your real smell rather than mask it. If you find this difficult, play it safe by only using the most minuscule amount.

Pheromones are released in abundance from the temples, just in front of your ears, behind your ears, armpits, elbow creases, behind the knees, between your toes, especially the smallest two, and between the fingers, especially between the little and ring fingers.

So if you're having problems hooking into pheromone situations with other people, try sniffing their temples to speed things up a bit.

Apply scent discreetly to tempular indentations, behind your ears, in your armpits, in your elbow creases, and behind your knees. Many women find it advantageous to sex-life activity to apply a small amount of their own vaginal secretion garnered during ovulation time, mixed in with the perfume of their choice.

Above all, avoid using scents that smell like fly spray (no brand names mentioned), deodorant that makes you smell like a men's locker room, or soap that makes you smell like a mortician or lab technician.

Importance of being comfortable with your own sexuality

If you're not, how can you be comfortable with someone else's? How can he/she be comfortable with yours? That's what makes sex uncomfortable, excessively coarse pubic hair and/or confined spaces notwithstanding.

To be truly comfortable with your sexuality, you have to truly accept all your strange little/not-so-little sexual quirks, and love yourself for them. Contrary to the biblical ethos, you have to be able to love yourself physically. And yes, I mean jerking off. Have a shower. Dry off. Get some nonrancid, preferably sexually sympathetic smelling massage oil, and in the privacy of your own room/bathroom, massage slowly down the front of your torso, spending luxurious moments teasing your breasts/manly chest and nipples, slowly stroking down over your belly to, you guessed it, your special place, i.e., genitals. Rub the oil gently into your genitals. Rub it up the inside of your thighs. Rub it into your asshole, your perineum, and scrotum, if you have one. Whisper sweet nonsense to yourself ("I'm so sexy, I love myself so much, I can't give myself enough pleasure"), then proceed to do just that (give yourself enough pleasure). And don't be ashamed afterward. Don't pretend you didn't just do that. Reassure yourself. Say something like, "It is good to engender pleasure in myself for myself. It is part of my ongoing sexual healing process," then have another shower if you need to and carry on as you were. If the sexual phase of the action can be completed satisfactorily without recourse to fantasy, i.e., with fully-present-in-the-moment pure sexual intelligence, then so much the better.

Good, now you've deepened your sexual relationship through comfort with yourself, opening the way for this to occur satisfactorily with an O.

But for the process to have true impact you need to develop the following attribute (in abundance).

Self-esteem

Tricky one, this. It comes and goes like a slippery fish, depending on previous (childhood) factors, the state of your health and energetic balance, time of month/year/life, as well as the state of health and energetic balance of the communication, sexual and otherwise, between you and Os.

But building and sustaining it runs along the lines of self-inculcated thought/belief patterns such as: "I was special/ unique/ worthy/valid/sweet-souled enough to have emerged from the Tao as a fully formed human being, so I am special/unique/worthy/ valid/sweet-souled enough to be desirable/attractive/irresistible to [suitable] others."

Somewhat of a mouthful, I know, but you can paraphrase it at will or just lift bits from it. For example, "I am desirable." (That's true.) Or, "I am a healthy sexual human being."

It's not the words of the affirmation, it's the essence that's important. You want/need/benefit from the feeling of sexual self-esteem you get when you believe it to be so.

Say, "I'm beautiful," and for one moment before the goblins come, feel your beauty. Good.

Now say, "I'm totally sexually desirable." Let yourself feel it. Good.

So when I say, "You beautiful sexy thing you," just say, "I know. Thank you."

The reflections of each other we see in the mirrors we hold up during the sharing of sexual love are the strongest. If you're coming to the sexual arena riddled with low sexual self-esteem, you'll transmit that to O, who'll respond either by feeling sexually inadequate or by becoming abusive/dominating. Either way, the energy between you will be unbalanced and so will how you feel about it afterward.

And never go into a sexual situation with somebody because you think they'll boost your self-esteem, because the way cause and effect work, you'll come out of it feeling worse.

Take your low self-esteem off with your socks/stockings. Come to the sexual arena proud to be who you are.

Inhibitions

Work toward being able to fully accept/love the entire range of sexual activities two (or more) people can enjoy with each other, in the natural expression of their naked selves.

This does not include learning to accept/love the use of equipment for pain infliction or bondage, special clothing, or the enforced sharing of vomit, piss, or shit. That's at your discretion.

But to feel easy with as great a range of sexual activity and expression as you can makes you more interesting/exciting as an O. It doesn't mean you have to lick everyone's asshole just to prove you're liberated. It just means that O can sense the depth of your experience, the lack of fear, and the feeling of confidence that engenders. Being a prude just isn't sexy. But as you know, being rude is.

Being rude

Being rude means literally being at one with the rudiments, i.e., the basic foundations, of life. That level of existence where you smell the vaginal secretion, taste the sperm, where you are connected fully and unashamedly to the roots of bioplasmic reality.

Rude in this context does not infer crude. Crude is cruddy, especially around the delicate environment of sexual love. Rude, on the other hand, is simply rude.

Importance of physical fitness, flexibility, suppleness, and stamina

It's obvious, unless you're into very lazy sex, that for it to be any good, you've got to be relatively fit, flexible, and supple so you can explore the full range of possible movement available to you without doing your back in, getting cramps in your legs, hurting your neck, fainting, or having a heart attack. And you need stamina, especially if you're a man, to sustain your adventure beyond the twenty-minute mark.

When your stamina is strong, your sex will be strong and leave you feeling strong afterward. When your stamina is lacking, your sex will be too and you'll feel even weaker afterward.

So get down on that floor and do those eighty-one push-ups and eighty-one sit-ups, lift those free-weights, do that power-yoga class, and run those three extra miles. Do something psychophysically enhancing every day so you're always in shape for that next telling moment when you take your clothes off.

Taking your clothes off

If you've got a routine sorted out, fine. If not, you may find the following sweeping generalizations, to which there are obviously many exceptions, quite useful.

First, be proud of who you are and how you appear. Even if, by conventional media-dictated standards, you think you're deficient (everyone does, at least occasionally). The reason for this is that once you're standing naked in front of O, there's nothing you can do to disguise yourself. So you may as well be proud of what you've got, because that's a lot sexier than looking/acting mealy-mouthed about it.

Second, be natural, without artifice. Don't try to look sexy as you disrobe, unless you're doing parody, of course, because it's immediately transparent and thus mildly embarrassing for any sensitive O, who automatically sees your insecurities (which is not usually sexy). There's nothing wrong with insecurities, unless you attempt to hide or disguise them, especially when doing a "sexy" undressing maneuver.

Third, maintain eye contact in a natural, unhostile sort of way, but not at the expense of losing balance while taking your pants off.

Fourth, don't be afraid to show your vulnerability. It's sexy to be who you are, even if your belly's a mite bloated, your ass a bit saggy, or your tits/willy a bit teeny.

Fifth, always take off the garments covering the top part of your body first, as it often tends to look top-heavy and slightly stupid to be wearing all your street paraphernalia with no pants/skirt.

Sixth (boys), take off your socks before taking off your pants and underwear, as standing there in socked feet and tighty-whities tends to make you look like a goon. You may find yourself and O helping/ripping each other out of your clothes. In these cases, it's perfectly permissible to help boys unhook bra straps, as this action doesn't generally come naturally. By the same token, boys must feel no compunction about asking girls to turn around so they can unhook the strap more easily. The important thing is to do whatever you do with authority.

The significance of movement

Sexual action requires movement. You're either moving a particular body part—your hand, your finger, your tongue, your lips, your genitals, your hips, your legs—or you're moving the whole shooting match in a series of unbroken, gyroscopic undulations.

How you move and where you're moving from (and to) are of the utmost relevance. How you move directly affects how your partner moves (that's obvious). So it isn't just a selfish thing we're into here.

Refocus your awareness away from exclusive concentration on tits and butts/cocks and biceps so that you become aware (mindful) of your own body movements from the inside. Feel your breath moving, tongue darting, hips grinding, arms entwining, from the inside; from that deepest part of you us romantics call your soul.

In that place you contact the mystery of your own creation. Many people are willing, even need/want, to undergo the contrived constriction of physical/emotional bondage and/or pain to reach here. That's how good it is. But you don't *need* to hurt or constrict yourself or others to reach it.

When in full sexual contact you activate this inner awareness of deepest mystery, and automatically transmit that awareness through your body and chi to your partner.

At the point where two souls meet during the sexual action, it is then possible to start mutually playing consciously with the energy between you to bring on the state of shared/solo sexual nirvana.

Sexual nirvana

Imagine the peak of the best/biggest/earth-shakingest orgasm, going on and on, like some huge, endless mountain plateau at an altitude of thirty-one thousand feet.

Now imagine that instead of this orgasm being genital-centered (genitocentric), i.e., occurring in your lowest Tan Tien (belly), it's occurring in your upper Tan Tien (center brain), with its roots rising up from deep within your loins, passing up through your middle Tan Tien (chest) like a controlled nuclear explosion, lighting up the inside of your brain.

Just beneath the crown of your head, up at the top of your brain, is a psychic region known as the Ni Wan (Nirvana) Peaks.

By use of the Big Squeeze technique [See *The Big Squeeze*, p. 117], and a bit of careful attention at the right moment, you will, with a surprisingly minimal amount of practice, be able to transport yourself, as if by psychic helicopter, to the loftiest heights of the Ni Wan Peaks, supported on a cushion of intense sexual ecstasy, there to sustain the experience for as long as you can bear it. (It's not always easy to stand on the mountaintop for extended periods. You need to build up resistance to the strong psychic winds you get up there.) Returning to your body when you've had enough is like being wafted down onto a feather bed. Once back down, you feel as though your brain has just been jet-washed and pumped full of concentrated light, as though your entire personality has been thoroughly gone over at the Chinese laundry and is now sparkling, shiny, and new. You have the irrefutable sensation that *everything* in/about your life is definitely OK.

When O is simultaneously, consciously engaged in doing this with you, the combined effect can be of such awesome synergetic impact that the two of you will be wobbly for days to come.

Why would you want to do this?

Because it's a Class A trip, there's nothing else on the open market to touch it, it leaves you feeling like a superhuman, and when you've been there once you'll be scrambling to get back.

The delicate mechanisms involved in triggering this supremely altered state are such that it doesn't always work. When you first start practicing, the initial occurrence ratio is about one in ten, but as with any new sport, the more you practice, the higher the frequency of successful missions.

As with all naturally attained altered states, you can't force it, but the method for attaining it is so simple and fool-friendly, that with self-patience even the most bumbling clod can get it. How much easier then for you.

Tempo

Whether you're just using the back of your hand to caress O's upper arm, or your entire body for high-velocity pump 'n' thrusting, always be conscious of the tempo you're moving at.

It is best to keep pulling your tempo back (to around 80 beats per minute), as tactile sensation is most easily assimilated/enjoyed slowly. When the action moves too fast, your nervous system doesn't have time to make any sense of the information; it becomes an itchy blur. And on top of that, if you do everything at your top speed of 2,323 miles an hour, you'll have no more to give when you need to accelerate for the climax, and will exhaust yourself and make your head spin.

Practice slowly, just like tai chi, to give yourself time to fully experience the sublime beauty of each tiny part of every movement, from deep within your Spirit Body. This is meditation in action, which is much easier to concentrate on when you slow yourself down.

What's the rush anyway?

Go from slow to fast and from fast to slow, allowing yourself ample time in medium too. Give the event dynamics.

The delicate mechanism which triggers sexual nirvana requires a slow tempo to set it off. Even a straightforward, mind-boggling orgasm is fourteen times stronger when achieved slowly (and approximately forty-eight times stronger when achieved in complete stillness).

But no matter how fast or slow the tempo of your external movement, your mind must always be kept on a slow turn (around 8 beats per minute) so you can assimilate what's happening and consciously remain with it. And the way you keep your mind turning at a slow tempo is to keep your breath slow. No more breathless panting like a dog, in other words. [See *Breathing*, p. 112.]

Alertness to signals

While remaining fully relaxed throughout, you must always remain alert to the signals of pleasure/displeasure O is giving off.

Don't wait for O to say, "That hurts," before you remove your heavy kneecap from her tit/your penetrating elbow from his balls.

Remember, this is a freestyle improvisational dance, where you respond to O and O to you, not just another opportunity for you to run through all your well-rehearsed act. So if you want spontaneous bliss to erupt from the Tao of the dance, be alert to the signals O is giving you, through facial expression, sound, and body movement.

Counting repetitions as meditation

This is of import mostly for the boys. You will notice in "The Sting" section of the handbook, dedicated to showing you what you actually do, that a certain amount of repetition is recommended with each move you make. The amount of repetition, though based on traditional and Wayward Taoist numerological values, is obviously arbitrary and intended only as an optional guide.

Counting repetitions is a good way to still/engage the monkey-mind and helps you remain fully present in the moment, possessed of clear sexual intelligence. Counting helps turn sex into meditation and is useful in counteracting the tendency to ejaculate by surprise [see below].

No longer needing to distract yourself with ugly thoughts to prevent premature ejaculation

This is also for the boys. By practicing fully-conscious-in-the-present-moment awareness during sex, making use of slow-tempo breathing, doing the Big Squeeze [see *The Big Squeeze*, p. 117], and counting repetitions, in addition to ceasing all movement and asking O to do likewise at crucial moments, and even pulling out when necessary, you will no longer need to use such schoolboy devices as imagining your grandmother taking a crap or reciting the subway map in your mind, in order to prevent untimely ejaculation.

The question of premature ejaculation

Again, this is mostly for the boys, but has obvious advantageous effects for girls too.

It would be more accurate to describe this phenomenon as "sudden surprise ejaculation." Even "untimely ejaculation" is imprecise. "Premature" and "untimely" imply a given time-phase during which it is ungentlemanly/unmanly to discharge your load.

"Surprise" is more precise, because that's exactly what happens. You have every intention of going on until she's at least come twice, or even of not coming at all, and you're doing fine, completely happy with what's going on, in full sexually intelligent awareness, breathing slowly, meditating like a copulating Buddha, when all of a sudden, she makes a moan or some unusual turn of hip, you are taken by the romance, and before you even know what's happened, you're on that irreversible rocket ride, which is going to lead to an inevitable squirt and shudder.

Never be ashamed of yourself for coming like that. It's your unbridled self having free rein. Delight in that. You're perfectly entitled to grow bored if it's something you find yourself indulging in frequently, but to be ashamed is like the sky being ashamed of itself when it rains on a sunny day. Shit happens.

Ejaculation occurs when you choose it to. The tricky thing is that the choice is made for you, as it were, by your own unconscious mind. That is, unless you consciously wrest this choice-making faculty away from it.

First, at the start of any serious action, make a conscious choice about how long you want to go on before you come, if at all.

Second, keep your breath-tempo slow. Panting speeds up your energy, heart rate, and mental activity. Breathing deeply and slowly, regardless of how fast or slow your body is moving, slows your mind, energy, and blood, which is essential for you to maintain full conscious choice of when and if to splurge.

Third, practice the Big Squeeze. [See *The Big Squeeze*, p. 117.]

Fourth, relax. [See *Relaxation*, p. 115.]

Fifth, practice inner alchemy. [See *Inner alchemy*, p. 124.]

Sixth, stop moving and, if necessary, request O to do the same, well before you begin the irreversible ascent.

Seventh, if you are with dick vaginally ensconced, pull back to the entrance, or, if necessary, out altogether. Timing must be accurate, however, because it's a real drag pulling out and then half-coming through a dribbling ejaculation before you've even got time to jerk yourself off.

And don't be hard on yourself (pun), if, even with all these techniques, you seem to lose the thread of consciousness as the goblins run interference on your mind, and you find yourself yet again ejaculating by complete surprise. It happens to (nearly) everyone from time to time.

It should be noted that you are far more prone to sudden surprise ejaculation attacks when your kidney energy is low, through illness, stress, extreme cold, or just basic exhaustion. Eat a knob of raw ginger every day and keep your kidneys warm, especially in the dread cold winds and damp of winter.

Naturally, it is preferable for O-girl to enjoy a good orgasm or several before boy-O comes, but essentially O-girl's orgasm is O-girl's responsibility, not boy-O's. Indeed, there are some women who are so in tune with their own sexuality that they come with full force as quickly as boy-O would like them to. And then there are others who know exactly how to make boy-O lose it and come too fast just so they can feel more powerful and in control. It obviously has a lot to do with the particular chemistry and dynamics of the situation at hand.

The most important thing is to be proud as you come, no matter when, and go with it fully, lending it your total emotional support. Because if you're going there anyway, you might as well enjoy it while it's happening. You can save your veiled/not-so-veiled mealy-mouthed excuses/apologies/justifications for later.

The mystery of chemistry

It could be the way O looks. It could be the way O smells. It could be the way O walks. It could be the way O talks. It could be anything. That's the point. It's a mystery.

It's either there or it isn't. There's nothing you can do about it. Sure, you can augment it by looking pretty/handsome (even pretty handsome), smelling good, washing behind your ears, acting groovy, even having a great personality, but you can't force chemistry.

Not that it should be ignored/dismissed on that account. It is essential to be perceptive to chemistry, and changes in levels thereof, in both initiatory and ongoing sexual scenarios.

Chemistry also fluctuates with a woman's menstrual cycle, usually increasing in intensity during the ovulatory phase.

In fact, there are many Taoists (Wayward and otherwise) who believe that the chemistry, i.e., juice, is supplied, regulated, and controlled exclusively by the woman, and that the man merely responds to her chemical output. [See *The significance of smell*, p. 59.]

Dynamics

Always be sensitive to the dynamics or context of the situation in which you find yourself embroiled with O.

It may be, for example, that O is really someone else's supposedly exclusive O, or that you are, and you and O are doing your experiments behind one or two other Os' backs, and that if you take the other Os out of the equation, the fire between you extinguishes.

It may be just a holiday romance, which simply doesn't travel well.

You may be an aristocrat, minor or otherwise, indulging in a bit of low-rent sex, which may work fine in the boudoir, but not at cocktails.

It may be that you only appreciate/desire O when you're feeling depressed/desperate/down, and when you're up and confident, you don't want to know O anymore.

It may work while you're part of a triangle but not when it's just the two of you.

It may work fine in the office but not, etc., etc.

It's all down to lighting, camera angle, set design, props, supporting actors and extras, and story line. In other words, the dynamics of the situation, which will determine how the outcome is affected/dictated by your perception. Dynamics, as the word implies, are constantly shifting, and remaining perceptive to their changing phases is like watching the weather forecast so you know what to wear tomorrow.

Are there such things as soul mates?

Yes. Momentarily at least. [See *Moments, series of*, below.]

Of course, there will be times in your life when your soul is at such and such a stage of evolution that you will look deep into the eyes of someone across a crowded room and recognize, in that flash of falling in love at first sight, your own self. Only it won't appear that way because you'll already be enamored of that person's form and thinking how you've just met your soul mate. And that person may well be feeling/thinking the same way about you.

And sure, it's possible you'll both spend the rest of your long and happy lives together, exclusively. But it's also possible you won't, and that when you've stopped being sentimental about it, you'll meet another soul mate with whom to share your magic moments.

It's quite possible, you see, that the soul is multifaceted and that you require a different soul mate to reflect that particular soul-facet currently on display. Who's to say? For with all the spiritual bullshit written about the soul over the years, no one actually knows the rules. It's all just been conjecture.

The main thing is to rejoice in the dynamism of every meeting between you and any soul mates who happen along your path down the Great Thoroughfare, without clinging to one particular form. No one is indispensable (when you get down deep enough).

Moments, series of

When you fantasize about your perfect soul mate engaged with you in your perfect romantic scenario, it is good to recall that what you fantasize is merely a moment or series of moments.

You picture him/her riding up on his/her horse and scooping you out of your own story line to a new and better movie, there to live in everlasting bliss till ye both die. It's a moment you're looking at.

It's helpful to remember this when your longing for one particular person is beginning to upset your digestion.

Is there a perfect mate?

You may well find yourself enjoying a perfect moment. You may even find yourself sharing it with a perfect mate. You may find, though, that a perfect mate from one shared magic moment of perfection is a damn lousy one when the magic changes, as magic usually does.

According to the immutable law of Yin and Yang, there's always a dark side to every story. If you can accept/love/welcome the dark side as much as the light in someone (and, of course, yourself), you can have that person as your perfect mate for a while, maybe even a long while, assuming he/she feels like playing too.

As long as you remember that, first, nothing and no one is in a static state of perfection. It would not only be impossible, but deathly dull to boot. And, second, that everything and everyone (including you) is absolutely perfect exactly as it/he/she is. Absolutely perfect, mate.

Dropping expectations

Have no expectations and you'll have no disappointments. Especially when it comes to love and sex with other people. If you can't manage that, at least be aware when you're building up expectations about someone, i.e., someone in a particular situation or series of situations with your good self. And remember that some expectations may coincide with their respective outcomes and some won't, so don't take it personally either way.

Never expect another human to behave in a particular way, even if he/she has behaved that exact same way 490 times before. Always factor the random into your picture.

Expecting someone to love you a certain way is a certain way to kill the way they love you.

By the same token, always, without fail, expect the very best for yourself and everyone else, from every situation in which you find yourself enmeshed. But do not cling to any pictures you subsequently conjure up regarding the outcome. Sow the seed, water the ground, but let the Tao take care of the tree growing.

So drop the expectation, handle the disappointment with grace and dignity when/if it comes, in full knowledge that you'll always get whatever you need for your healthy growth, and let life surprise you a little.

The case for
serial monogamy

It's a bit like a game of poker.

You meet O. You go through the phases. I want you, I want you. I love you, I love you. I hate you, I hate you. I'm bored. I gotta get outta here. I want someone else. And so on. Maybe you move through the phases *real* slow like they used to in the old days, so that you die before you get to wanting someone else.

Probably you don't, though. (Maybe you're already bored but don't want to admit it.)

Maybe your love, wisdom, bonding mechanism, and communication skills are so strong (mutually) that there's no way you'd even consider any other O.

But maybe they're not, and with the general exponential acceleration and intensification of human behavior at the present time, along with the media-inspired push toward exploring the proliferation of choices available in your personal activities, you perhaps get restless after the communication between you and O inevitably goes pear-shaped, as it will from time to time, and start desiring other Os.

Maybe you suppress/self-deny these desires for sentimental/economic/social-status reasons. Maybe you meet someone (these things happen), and you can't suppress the desire.

Metaphysically speaking, we come together in loving union with other Os to help each other transform. We do this by providing mirrors for each other, which reflect both the nicer aspects and the smellier ones.

Maybe you've had all the reflection of that particular aspect of yourself you can take for now. Maybe it's time to take another module in the course.

Maybe it's entirely astrological.

But there comes a time in many modern lovers' lives when they simply have to move on, to do the dance with someone new.

In this respect, many modern lovers like to think of themselves as serial monogamists. This entails making some kind of spoken or unspoken/implied agreement/contract as regards exclusivity rights. This constitutes what is popularly and confusingly termed a "commitment." That is, you bind yourself, wittingly or unwittingly, to upholding your sexual exclusivity agreement, or at least faking it, until you (or O) declare that you wish to discontinue. The consequences of that depend on the social, legal, financial, and moral factors appertaining to your particular situation at that time.

It is quite common for there to be a cross-fade period, as you attempt to fade one story out and a new one in simultaneously, just like any good DJ would. Even though this affords moments at which there is likely to be more than one other person involved in your sexual activities, it still seems to fall within the popular definition of serial monogamy and is simply referred to knowingly as the crossover phase. [See *All is fair in love and war*, p. 101.]

It's all just a play in the mind
meaning?

I mean, you're standing in the hallway of your house. Your partner/husband/regular O is out playing with your children, and you're saying good-bye to a guy with whom you're conducting a secret romance. Nothing's happened (yet), just lots of talking (talking, talking, talking). You invited him around just so you could see him in the context of the familiar. You wanted to tease yourself with the juxtaposition. You sat together, talking, drinking tea, not touching, but penetrating and caressing each other with your eyes. So beautiful. The sexual tension is building to the point that it's nearly unsustainable. You long to hold each other. You don't. Both of you feel nervous about your partner and children coming home. You're loving the nervousness. The adrenaline is your addiction.

It's come time for your auric lover to go. At the door, you suddenly find yourself in each other's arms. Holding, feeling, hands moving over your back. You're going, you're going, melting, and your lips touch, mouths hungry to kiss, to devour. His tongue darts delicately between your lips just for an instant, then you turn your head away. Because you have to. Because you know instinctively that it's not right/too soon. But you're still holding on to each other. Then he moves away, you open the door, your eyes locked on to each other's, producing an almost visible field between you, of love, desire. You feel wet. You close the door behind him and walk down the hallway, and as you walk, you come.

It wasn't the action of walking, moving your legs, that made you come.

It wasn't him who made you come.

It was the play in your mind, the intensity of entertaining the idea of doing something "wrong," the tease of feeling his body against yours, of feeling his sexual essence, just fleetingly.

It was all just the play in your mind.

The case for nonserial monogamy

I don't know, do people still do that?

They say certain whales do it but who knows what they get up to down there in the depths. Some swans too, but people, no cheating, ever?

I've heard stories of things like this, especially among the generation born between World Wars One and Two, but have never had it verified whether this included or was nullified by extra-monogamous affairs on the sly. I'm sure, at least in my more sentimental moments, there are couples who've been together since they were both virgins, and who've stayed together through thick and thin, without ever so much as a furtive longing glance at anyone else, who've never strayed even momentarily with the guy fixing the kitchen, the girl at reception, or their partner's best friend. I'm sure there must be couples like that. Maybe you're part of one yourself. But the way things are, you may be part of someone's floating harem.

The case for the floating harem

The floating harem, as opposed to the traditional, fixed harem, as in a building full of concubines and eunuchs, is becoming more and more popular among modern lovers. Or, more precisely, more and more modern lovers are owning up to the fact that they informally maintain a floating harem.

Though traditionally it was the man who kept a harem of women, it is now just as common for a woman to keep a harem of men. Polygyny and polyandry, though not in the formal sense, are fast becoming the preferred mode for many modern lovers.

Some harem keepers are honest about it (some of the time). Most aren't (most of the time). Even with themselves.

It's impossible to get all the stimulation and reflection that you want/need, all the time, from just one person, unless that person is so multifaceted/talented that you never grow weary of him/her, even after you've heard that person's repertoire fifty times, however enlightened/generous/self-contained you may be.

It's impossible to *always* get the exact kind of sexual hit you want from just one person, unless you're both extremely inventive, flexible, forgiving, and incredibly sexy (to each other all the time).

So people get up to things with other people, with other Os, they shouldn't (according to their nebulous moral code).

Sure you can love more than one person at a time. You can love ten if you're relaxed enough, and if you space them out visit-wise enough.

Sometimes it takes a month for you to get the desire for someone back strongly enough after the last time, to actually act it out with them again. Sometimes it takes a day. So you space the time spent with each haremee accordingly.

I'm not saying it's right or wrong. I'm just saying it's the way it is (for some of the modern lovers some of the time). So now you know.

Monogamy requires skilled mental/emotional acrobatics from both parties. You see someone you fancy, and have to deftly and swiftly file them under never-never before your mind has time to go into fantasy/desire mode. Sometimes you don't catch it in time and you're off in another one of your silent head-spins. But if monogamy sits well with you, if that's the way you choose to make sense of the nonsense, then that's what you do.

Polygamy and so-called serial monogamy also require feats of mental/emotional acrobatics, making sure you don't get the names mixed up in bed.

Whatever blows your hair back, but the important thing is to be honest with yourself. [See *Honesty as an aphrodisiac*, p. 89.]

Importance of flirting

Flirting, the traditional Parisian sport, predating *j'ai allé*, is essential to your emotional well-being. A beautiful flower in the garden will probably not wilt if no one pays it much attention. But you're not a flower, and unless you are completely enlightened and totally free of all desire, in which case you shouldn't be bothering yourself with this material, you need attention from people you find attractive feeding back to you, with a darting glance or a silken word, that you're attractive to them too. It reminds you of your sexual, i.e., creative, power, it lifts your spirits, and if it's with someone really dishy it makes you feel damn fine.

Flirting often leads to real mischief, but it doesn't have to. Indeed, the art of the sophisticated flirt is that of both parties coming away feeling as though they just had the best fuck of their lives without even having touched each other. It's all in the eyes.

Often just knowing you could have a little love story is enough. It has to be. You'll never find time to fuck all the women/men. It's a bottomless pit.

But flirting is good for your health and good for your self-esteem, which, in turn, is good for any O or Os you spend your time with.

Do not be put out if you catch an O of yours flirting with someone else. Be happy. You wouldn't want to be with an ugly flower no one else wanted. And if an O of yours is so insecure that he/she gets nasty/possessive when the person watches you flirt harmlessly with other people, send him/her to a therapist or back to the caves.

In fact, it is important for the health of a long-term arrangement to observe your O flirting with others. It reminds you of the person's worth.

Obviously there's flirting and flirting, and I'm not for a moment suggesting you indulge in vulgar displays of lust/naked passion. No, always be subtle and discreet and remember your manners, i.e., always give some visual clue to your/their partner, where appropriate, that it's just a harmless flirt you're having, with no malice aforethought involved. Never flirt so hard/obviously that you make a fool of yourself or them (unless you want to make a fool of yourself . . . or them).

If both parties to the flirt are unencumbered by any exclusivity agreement, imaginary or otherwise, with any other lover, imaginary or otherwise, or if one or both parties is desirous of a personnel change, flirting effectively is likely to lead to seduction.

Nature of seduction

Seduction, from the Latin *seducere*, means to lead someone unto yourself.

So how good you are at seduction depends on how good you are at leading.

There are many styles of leadership/seduction, from the outright fascistic to the wheedlingly emotionally manipulative, but the Taoist style is to lead from behind.

Always lead as if you're following.

Seduction is tantamount to putting a spell on someone, strong enough to lead them away from their own story line/agenda, toward yours for a while. This is obviously easier to accomplish when your seductee signals that he/she is willing to play along.

The Wayward Taoist approach to leading from behind is to simply, humbly, yet confidently make your desires known to all relevant parties and then let go (and wait). If it is in accord with the Tao of the situation, i.e., for the highest good of all concerned, and by the free will of all concerned, what you want will happen of itself in the appropriate manner at the appropriate/divinely appointed moment.

If it doesn't, forget it and move on, with the confidence that when one trap door closes a better one always opens (so watch out).

Obviously I'm aware that everybody has their own particular seduction routine/style/technique, which varies somewhat in tone and delivery, depending on whom you're using it with, but whichever style you're adopting, the most effective way is to say what you want, honestly and clearly, without expectation, embarrassment, shame, or fear of rejection/humiliation, and then stand back and wait for as long as it takes for your seductee to make that idea their very own (if they want to), so they feel like it's their story line they're living and not yours. Then if they come back with an "OK, big boy/girl, your place or mine," you simply follow, as if it was their idea all the time. This is leading/seducing from behind. (At least that's the way it always worked for this Wayward Taoist.)

Boundaries and personal/ interpersonal space

A delicately poised love affair is one in which both parties recognize, understand, and respect the invisible personal boundaries of the other, and so maintain clarity in the interpersonal space between them.

Looks good on paper, but will it work?

For about as long as each of you is clear about your own boundaries and where they lay. The extent to which either of you is confused about your own boundaries is the extent to which the interpersonal space between you is clouded by confusion.

Only when the boundaries are (relatively) clear between you can you engender a space for mutual trust, requisite to anything from an erotic moment to a lifetime partnership.

Trust

It's not a matter of whether you trust O, it's a matter of whether you trust yourself (to be OK) being intimately/sexually involved with O.

Always trust all Os, whether newly met or Os you've lived with for the past thirty-nine years, to be nothing more than human. And that includes all human "failings"/foibles, including dishonesty, deceit, perfidy, and treachery, including being able to look you straight in the eye and say, "I didn't," when they did, without twitching or displaying any other telltale body-language signs to the contrary. And this doesn't apply only to other people. It applies to you too.

Trust is when the feeling in your belly is settled and warm, so you feel safe and comfortable with that particular O. (Because that's all everyone wants, to feel safe and comfortable around someone, even if safe and comfortable is composed of dangerous and scary, as it usually is—we're all adrenaline addicts.) You "trust" them on an animal/instinctive level, to honor and respect the unique expression of divine perfection you personally represent, i.e., you trust yourself to be able to express your divine perfection with them. As soon as that stops, it's time for negotiation/quitting.

It's also about each of you trusting yourselves to be able to create an appropriate environment/setting/context in which to act out your erotic moments together in a way you'll hopefully both be proud of afterward.

This state is achieved through communication.

Communication

Communication is the act of consciously sending signals, through the media of voice and body/body part movement, to another person, in this case an O, for the purpose of getting what you want.

The first time you did this was the first time you screamed to be fed and someone stuck a tit/teat in your mouth. From then on it was just a matter of refining your style.

The words you speak/shout/scream/sing/chant carry the idea across the interpersonal space between you and O. That's just a percentage of the action though. The *sound* of your voice, affected by the level of relaxation/tension in your skull, throat, thorax, and diaphragm, is what substantiates your words and is what makes the difference between genuine/authentic verbal communication and that of, say, a politician or used car salesperson.

It's about where your voice is coming from. If you're so twisted up inside with the discomfort of the moment that you've forgotten to breathe properly and are hence constricted in the upper body, your voice will only come from your throat. The vibrations it carries as you vocalize will therefore only find resonance in the throat of the recipient. For your words to hit home, however, they have to resonate all the way down, deep into the listener's gut, the lower TT. To make this happen, *you* have to speak from *your* lower Tan Tien. The sound has to originate in your belly. Then what you say comes from your core and your words ring true. That's how people instinctively know when you're lying (if they're quick and in tune enough to notice); they don't feel your words resonate in their belly.

When you wish to conduct authentic dialogue with O—the type of communication necessary for one erotic moment, or a whole lifetime's series of them (as in long-term scenarios)—do so with a relaxed body, arms and legs uncrossed, to make you energetically available, eyes steady and straight, maintaining full eye contact at all times, and supporting your words with adequate amounts of breath so the sound comes out from deep inside your core.

(And everything'll be just fine. Just fine.)

It's the essence you communicate that creates the context/setting/environment for the erotic moment to occur, not the silk sheets, candles, incense, ambient jazz, perfume, or doing funny things with your tongue and facial expressions.

But don't get too hung up on it. It's all just a play in your mind.

Honesty

We live in a demented loony bin, in which it is a major achievement to manage moments of honesty with yourself, let alone trying to manage moments of honesty with someone else. To be true to yourself, about your motivations and intentions with regards to O, is your first obligation, for to attempt to be *truly* honest with O, verbally speaking, is impossible. The picture's simply too big.

Obviously, the ideal, to which we all aspire in our dreamier moments, is to always be fully honest with O, and for O to respond in kind. But as you may know from bitter experience, this is rarely, if ever, the case.

You disseminate information selectively. You even recall information selectively to yourself. During most "honest" dialogue, you're going crazy in the edit suite. Take note of all the outtakes next time you have a so-called honest chat with O. You will probably find the ratio of what comes out of your mouth to what ends up on the cutting room floor is somewhere in the region of 1:10, if that. (And I'm talking about being really honest with yourself here.)

However, that's fine. Even the moon is not obliged to show you her dark side. Honesty is relative. For everything you say, there's something you don't. It couldn't be otherwise; if it were, you'd spend your whole time saying things and O would have died of boredom before you'd made your point.

To open the possibility for self-honesty, you have to develop insight, which can be achieved through meditation, therapy, other sorts of sensitivity training, and simply spending periods of time alone to find out who you really are, what you really believe, and what you really, really want.

Honesty as an aphrodisiac

As long as you remember honesty is only relative, it's fine to use it as an aphrodisiac.

When you and O haven't been getting along too well, and you're holding back on communicating what's wrong for fear of rocking the boat, and the sex dries up because you feel cramped in your spirit, and you carry on like that until your soul gets uncomfortable enough to not care about rocking the boat any longer, and maybe Mercury comes out of retrograde, and you start to gush, and it all starts coming out, and somehow, miraculously, you seem to resolve it together, don't you find you have the best fucks? It's because you feel free again, unburdened of that weight of dishonesty in your brain, like any self-respecting animal should.

Dishonesty

There's only one thing you can say about dishonesty, other than we all know we shouldn't indulge in it, but do anyway (from time to time)—sometimes it's expedient.

Ideally, every interaction between you and O will be far sexier if you can be totally honest with each other all the time about absolutely everything, and I mean everything, without fail. This will not happen, however, because as you have already found out, sometimes it's expedient to be dishonest. I mean—lie.

If O's on the way to the gym and she asks, "Do you think my ass looks fat today?" and you have the guts to reply, "A bit, but it's nice," she then has the opportunity to set about changing that at the gym, if she wishes. If, however, the same question is asked just before O is leaving for an important presentation/meeting/social engagement and you know there's nothing she can do about her muscle tone right now, you answer, "No, your ass is beautiful." Well, don't you?

You know you're lying. She knows you're lying. You know she knows you're lying. And she knows you know she knows you're lying, but it's the sound she wanted to hear. It was the expedient thing to do in the situation if you wanted to avoid a nonsensical contretemps. And, of course, the same thing would apply if you asked her if she thought your dick was too small (any time—except if you're setting off for some penis enlargement surgery). Talking of which . . .

Is my dick too small?

(All brothers who are hung like donkeys need not fuss themselves over this item, except to snigger or deride if they so choose.)

Of course, sometimes your dick will be too small, and sometimes, hopefully usually, it won't. It all depends on the respective anatomy (and expectations) of you and O.

If an O-girl has an elephant-size vagina, her boy-O will more or less need an elephant-size dong to satisfy her, at least while inside her. If the woman is horse-sized, an elephant-size man is still good, a horse-size man will be perfect, a dog-size man not so perfect, and a rabbit-size man no good at all. If an elephant-size woman goes with a rabbit-size man, it's just stupid.

You get my point? It's nothing to be taken personally. Most male genitals apparently fall within the mid-range, so most of the time most of the people will mostly fit each other, more or less, probably.

So size does matter. Not as much as whether the world erupts into nuclear war, or whether a displaced refugee child gets anything to eat tonight, but it does matter. Just like good looks matter.

It wasn't meant to be fair. (And I'm not talking as a donkey. As previously stated, I'm a confirmed medium.)

However, you must always maintain perspective. It may make you blush and feel humiliated to be told by O that your cock's too small for her, but humiliation's only humiliation. It won't kill you unless you want it to. Remember that many women have the best sex of their lives with other women, who have absolutely no penis at all. Sex is all a play in the mind. Overwhelming pleasure can be given through your hands, lips, and tongue, as you know.

The real problem with size is the importance boys attach to it in terms of measuring their overall worth.

Dishonesty as an aphrodisiac

Just as honesty can be used as an aphrodisiac, so can dishonesty. Sometimes knowing that you have information about yourself and/or your doings, which if divulged to O would be temporarily devastating, gives you a sense of power. And that can be a turn-on.

Protecting O from the devastation you can potentially unleash through disclosure may make you feel compassionate and caring in a perverse sort of way. And that can be a turn-on.

Sometimes even the confusion in your twisted brain about it all can be a turn-on.

Twisted or not, it happens. Dishonesty can be an aphrodisiac.

It is simply good to realize this and to notice it if it should arise at some time or other, so you can forgive yourself. If you see a recurring pattern, consider spending time with an experienced therapist or healer (in a professional context).

Everyone's responsible for
their own experience here

You're not a victim. We all, at soul-level, create our own realities. Make an exception for children, i.e., those under the legal age, those suffering from severe mental disorders, and those who are otherwise physically incapable of defending themselves. Otherwise, whatever experience you manifest, with whomever, you manifest for yourself.

He didn't *make* you feel so horny you couldn't help yourself, *you* did. *She* didn't break your heart, *you* did. Or at least you gave her your heart to break, which you should never have done anyway. Give your love, not your heart. Love is infinite. Your heart isn't. You need it. [See *The nonsense of breaking people's hearts*, p. 238.]

What you experience is your responsibility.

Coming to the sexual arena as a victim sends a twisted message to O and you'll get a twisted experience.

Coming to it empowered by taking full responsibility for yourself makes you damn sexy and your subsequent experience will reflect that.

Manners, discretion,
and confidentiality

No matter who you're with or what you're doing together, always remember your manners.

Manners means waiting till O goes to the bathroom before you turn your head to look at that man/woman at the other table in the restaurant.

Manners means treating O with utmost respect at all times, just as you would a reigning king or queen or any other visiting foreign dignitary. Open doors, pull back bedsheets, pass the tissues, don't piss on the toilet seat, or spit on the floor, etc., etc. Remember that you lend whatever quality there is to the situation. Treat the situation well and it'll treat you well in return.

Manners means maintaining confidentiality about the secret/sacred things you and O get up to. Not just to keep them sacred, but to avoid later embarrassment when O finds out you've been telling the story to everyone in town.

Manners means discretion. Avoid giving secrets away about other people's private doings, even if those doings were done to you. You can tell stories of your escapades if you must, and most of us do from time to time, just don't mention any names. Got that?

Falling in love

Falling in love is like falling off a log. You've simply lost your balance momentarily.

You meet someone. They fit all your criteria, one way or another (all things considered). You go, "Wow." Casting session over. You've got your leading lady/man.

State of wow goes on while you build up a hugely positive (unbalanced) picture of O, complete with reworked story line to suit the actor, and proceed to project that fantasy onto O. At the same time you ignore or justify any traits, habits, and/or physical deficiencies not to your liking; after all, nobody's perfect (you say).

State of wow starts to diminish as soon as you see O's dark, all-too-human side is possibly more than you're able/willing to accommodate. This sometimes coincides with the third or fourth time you have sex (make love), when one or the other starts trying to fuck with the boundaries a little.

State of wow is over. (You hate to admit it but it's true.)

At this point, if you've got your wits about you and are not too blinded by your own agenda, you may discern exactly the way the power struggles are going to go, exactly the way you're going to drive each other mad, and exactly the way you'll have to compromise yourself to maintain the status quo.

If you're honest with yourself, you'll be able to make a free choice. Do I stay or do I go?

But it's hard to make that choice freely because you've fallen off your log and haven't got back on yet. You've made an investment of passion, fantasy-time, real-time, and energy. It's hard to kiss that good-bye. In any case, you've started to get addicted to this O and the story you've woven around him/her. And as with any addiction, you begin to kid yourself that you wouldn't be able to get along without it. So you start to cling. (And that's when the possessiveness kicks in and the insecurities loom large.)

So now you either gird your loins and engineer an appropriate ending, probably building up a watertight case against O to justify your destructive wishes. Or you stick around and pretend most of the time, and probably get married.

Or you get lucky and it turns out you're both intelligent, wise, loving, and compatible enough to sort it through and grow into a deeper state of love together. (Big shout to all long-term lovers!)

Mostly the wow stage of falling in love lasts one hormonal phase of three months, but with practice many modern lovers can get the whole thing over and done with in three days, often not even having to have sex, thus saving weeks, months, and even years of possible confusion and agitation, so they can carry on with their busy schedules and not mess up too many marketing plans, etc.

Falling in love is a lovely drug, and the more you do it the more you realize it's all just play in the mind. Just play in the mind.

Which isn't to say you shouldn't enjoy/cherish/value the loving at-
tachment(s) you have formed or will form in the future. Just that
maybe you learn to stop making movies in your head about people
and let the real movie that's been going on all the time anyway unfold on its own, without you getting in the way too much with your
expectations and agendas.

Love with all your heart, desire with all your loins, but don't fall
off your log, not for anyone. You'll do them/you no good like that.

Integrity/lack of

Integrity is the elusive quality you discern in someone when
they're all joined up with themselves—someone who is conversant
with all their aspects or subpersonalities, i.e., is integrated with
themselves, including all the mad bits.

It has nothing to do with being/acting perfect. It's to do with
knowing yourself and understanding/appreciating whichever role
you're playing at the time.

Integrity is not a constant state, it's fluid. We move in and out
of it continually, especially in our dealings with others, and especially with Os.

The trick to having integrity in the moment, for that is the best
you can hope for, is to keep bringing your awareness back to the
breath. Simple as that. Breathe.

As you bring your mind back to the breath, you automatically
and instantly regroup (all your subpersonalities). You become
aware of your three TTs, and as you do, O will experience you as
having integrity. Only then do your sexual encounters with O
come from a deep/true enough "place" inside you to have validity
and hence truly satisfy.

When you're out of integrity, i.e., displaying a lack of integrity/

integration, your energy (chi) is scattered and fragmented, and the outcome will be a scattered and fragmented sexual experience, leading to yet more confusion and difficult phone calls.

Fidelity

Fidelity comes from the Latin, *fides*, meaning faith. The word is also intimately related to the Latin, *fidere*, to trust.

In relation to your dealings with Os, it means remaining faithful in your heart both to the spirit of the agreement between you, and to the original loving intention toward O.

In fact, you're not faithful to O, you're faithful to the agreement between you.

Idealized fidelity is when you delude yourself into believing O never entertains desire for other Os. Realized fidelity is when you instinctively trust O to always have your best interests at heart, no matter what she/he gets up to when you're not around.

The only true fidelity is having faith in love, regardless of the twists and turns and personnel changes it takes you through.

Fidelity is something that happens of itself when the conditions are right. You can't force it. Attempting to remain faithful to someone, and/or to maneuver them into being faithful to you, causes more confusion than a self-assessment tax bill.

Remaining faithful to the love you feel for someone, and to the intention for them to flower and prosper, no matter what, is taxing on your good nature from time to time, but at least it makes sense.

Demanding fidelity is like laying claim to someone's soul. You can't possess another person. You can't even take possession of yourself most of the time. You can't possess someone's love, someone's desire.

You can't possess anything (for long). All you can do is trust.

Breathe, be fully present in the moment, and trust. Trust life/yourself to bring you all the love and sustenance you need. Trust life to bring the same to O. Be faithful to that.

Incidentally, Fido, the faithful dog, derives his name from fidelity.

Loyalty

Originating from the Latin, *lex*, meaning law, hence legal and loyal, loyal implies sticking to the rules of the situation, i.e., upholding the laws of the land, as in sticking by your king/queen.

Be loyal to the laws of your inner king/queendom, i.e., be true to yourself. Be true to the love you feel. Be true to the desire you feel.

Be true to the people you love (as much/often/fully as you can) and stick by them in times of need (as much/often/fully as you can).

Be loyal to the idea of people being able to live together in peace and mutual respect (for life) one day.

Be loyal to the natural laws of cause and effect which state that what's for ye won't pass ye by (and what's for O won't pass O by either).

Above all, be loyal to the love between you.

Treachery

Carefully pulling down the zipper of your lover's pants, gently and full of expectant awe of the phallic mystery, taking hold of his swelling erection in your dainty hand, slowly dropping to your knees and licking first the underside, then the top, then almost shyly putting your lips over the glans, parting them to allow his erection to fill your mouth, moving now to draw it in deeper, faster, and more confidently as you hold the shaft and suck with hunger. He feels your hunger. He feels your heat. He feels overwhelmed by the acute intensity of the situation. He comes suddenly and furiously. You swallow. You go home, kiss your husband on the cheek (you avoid the lips in case he smells a rat). "Good day?" "Yes, darling, and you?"

That's treachery.

Been there? Ever/yet?

Happens all the time. Obviously you wouldn't know it because we're all such good actors. And we delude ourselves that the grand charade is what's actually going on around here. But mostly it's not. That's why it's a charade. **Nothing is exactly how it appears.**

There will be times when even you may find yourself engaged in some more or less minor/major treachery toward one you love/have loved. If this should occur, rather than berate yourself, simply observe, acknowledge, and accept without judging yourself, as in, there I go again being treacherous. In this instance, if you're really honest with yourself, you might actually admit that, secretly, you enjoy being treacherous. Maybe that's why you do it.

I'm not advocating treachery here. I'm simply stating that it happens from time to time and that nothing constructive will be achieved by your committing hari-kari over it. Observe yourself doing it. Marvel at your Machiavellian capabilities and forgive yourself. Then love the person against whom you've just committed your treachery even more. (That's the challenging part.) Just love more (never less) and allow the theater to unfold as it will. Then go upstairs and wash your mouth out with soap and water (kidding).

Deceit

Do you deceive yourself? Do you deceive yourself constantly? Do you deceive yourself that all is well as you eat your breakfast, while a hundred thousand refugees, regular people like you and me, slept in a field in the snow last night? Do you deceive yourself that everything will be all right once you've got the mortgage/car/credit card/tax bill paid off? Do you deceive yourself that your personal existence has vast universal significance? Do you deceive yourself that you're going to be around like this forever? Do you deceive yourself that nasty things only happen to people you don't know? Do you deceive yourself that you never lie or in any other way break the/your so-called moral code? Do you deceive yourself that the sun sets and rises, when you know all along that it's just the earth rotating on its axis that causes the illusion of day and night? Do you deceive yourself that O isn't doing it/thinking about doing it with someone else from time to time? Do you deceive yourself that you're not deceiving O? Do you even deceive yourself that you're not deceiving yourself?

If not, you're enlightened.

The human capacity for self-deception is limitless. Without it we would probably be unable to survive daily life. Which is not to justify it, just to say that that's how it is.

How then could you be other than deceitful once or twice, at least, in your dealings with others, especially an intimate O?

Perhaps you've been thinking all week how you want to get out of this story line you've been sharing with O. O looks up from the pillow. "Have you had enough of this?" she asks. "No, of course not," you reply. Deception.

"Did you fancy that guy you were talking to tonight?" O means the beautiful hunky boy with the footballer's thighs, athlete's ass, and builder's biceps over whom you were secretly salivating at the party earlier. "Him? No, of course not. I love *you*," you reply, so innocently you even believe it yourself. Deception.

Maybe you just had sex with O. Maybe you weren't fully there for it. Your mind was wandering, remembering some stuff you have to do tomorrow, thinking about that girl/boy you bumped into at lunch, assessing the quality of the sex with O and deciding it was getting a bit old. "I love making love with you. Did you enjoy that?" she/he suddenly asks, piercing through your postorgasmic reverie. "Yes, it was beautiful," you say. Deception.

So what? you may rejoin.

So what exactly. Why make such a fuss about all the deception that potentially goes on (in any/every O to O situation). Accept deceit as an essential, unavoidable part of the play. At least don't deceive yourself about that, modern lover. Not even for a minute.

Lying/denying

Even the greatest gurus have admitted that sometimes it is expedient to lie. Sure it's smelly, but it's a fact of life.

If you've been having an illicit liaison and O's suspicion has been aroused, and providing you're pretty sure O has no hard proof and you wish to continue your present arrangement with O for a while longer without rocking the boat, when O confronts you with it, some wise masters/mistresses say: deny, deny, deny.

They tell you to remember it like a mantra: deny, deny, deny.

If you go this route, you have to be strong about it. Play the role with full conviction, and take responsibility for the psychic confusion that will inevitably result for both you and O.

This wisdom probably dates back to ancient Paris, where husbands and wives, mistresses and lovers, evolved a highly workable and sophisticated romance system (with only the odd crime of passion or two cropping up from time to time).

As an experiment in Wayward Taosim, however, you could try an alternative approach. Next time you're confronted by O for a correctly suspected sexual misdemeanor, simply admit it and see what happens next.

I'm not saying one approach is superior or inferior to another, though obviously the less lies you have to sustain, the more energy you'll have available for other possibly more enjoyable things (such as honest dialogue, for instance).

Ideally, respect yourself enough to respect Os enough to allow them to make their choices based on truth rather than lies.

Realistically, acting/pretense is as much an essential element of the game as catharsis from your core and being real. It's inevitable from time to time.

The important thing is to avoid lying and denying to yourself when you *know* something's true (you naughty thing you).

All is fair in love and war

I don't know which heartless beast first coined this axiom, but it's true.

Obviously we attempt to stick to the rules of the Geneva Convention, or at least be seen to be sticking to them. But every lover has his/her secret stash of chemical/biological weaponry, which the lover would use if pushed.

War is not fair. Love is not fair. That's the way it is. Why did you expect fairness? Where did this idea of fairness come from? Life is not fair. Life is fierce. Drop any expectations of fairness immediately to avoid any further pain of disappointment.

We each of us create our own realities. Accept that and accept full responsibility (from your end) for everything that transpires between you and O from here on in. Forget about fairness. All is fair in love and war.

This does not, however, mean that you should feel fine about acting like a heartless asshole with your lovers. Always do whatever you do with love, respect, compassion, and kindness (if you can manage it).

Being friends

Unless you're into pain and punishment, why would you want to share deep sexual/spiritual/intimate love with someone who's your enemy? Surely it's better to do that with a friend.

Old-fashioned lovers tended to differentiate between friends and prospective/actual lovers.

Modern lovers tend to regard people they like as potential/actual friends, whether or not they are or could be lovers.

Alliances and friendships between people where mutual sexual attraction is latent or active often lead to explorations along sexual lines at some time or another. While it is true that the aftermath of such explorations may result in temporary or permanent mutual discomfort, it is also true that they sometimes result in profoundly important ongoing liaisons.

Not that Os who are friends let you down any less than Os who aren't.

Friends let you down from time to time. Accepting that is part of enjoying fruitful friendships. **People disappoint. That's part of the system. People also delight. Hang on to neither. Expect both.**

And don't for a moment be fooled when he/she says, "I just want to be your friend," because nine times out of ten, it's bullshit.

(They're just betting on lulling you into a false sense of security and *then* pouncing.)

Commitment

You can commit yourself to be friends with someone for the rest of your life (providing they don't do anything to disappoint you beyond your disappointment threshold level).

You can, if you're extremely yogically advanced or highly imaginative/unimaginative, also commit yourself to finding one O attractive, exclusive of any others, for the rest of your life. However, you may find it problematic at times.

It makes perfect sense, if you've been in love with an O exclusively, every day, for the past twenty years, to say, "I've been in love with you exclusively, every day, for the past twenty years." But does it make any sense if you say to an O you've just met, "I promise to be in love with you exclusively, every day, for the next twenty years"?

(Not to me.)

Commit yourself to maintaining an open heart to every friend you make/have (including your lover[s]), and not turning any friend out of your heart/love until you die. Start by cracking that one and move on to more mind-boggling/detailed forms of commitment later.

Sex with strangers in confined spaces

From time to time, as a modern lover, you may find yourself with a relative stranger engaged in random acts of unbridled mutual expression of sexual love, i.e., you may find yourself fucking/suck-ing someone in a plane/train/club toilet or public telephone booth, for instance.

While this may be fun for you both at the time, you may also find it leaves you with a funny taste in your mouth.

The kind of compulsion that leads you into a confined space with a stranger can be interestingly transformed simply by bringing some love into the equation. Rather than watching yourself acting out scenes from a pornographic movie, see yourself engaged with another human being, one of your spiritual brothers/sisters, in the sharing of sacred sexual energy. Have compassion for them and yourself. Transform the toilet into a Taoist temple (Holy Mount Pu) with your love.

You may find, however, that this internal reframing action dampens your initial ardor somewhat. You may find yourself ask-ing, "What the fuck am I doing here?" Then again you may not.

Either way, the vast importance of the following cannot be un-derstated.

The vast importance of condoms

Because all the evidence points to high general levels of deceit (self-deceit and O-deceit), it is probably prudent to expect that no O can remain sexually monogamous, exclusively with you for as long as your exclusivity agreement runs, without even once slip-ping up.

It is probably far saner to assume that O is doing it behind your back from time to time, if your mind can stretch to that.

Not that I'm wishing that on you or encouraging you to be

paranoic. I'm just talking bottom lines and having your ass covered in the hopefully unlikely event of your being unwittingly deceived.

Hence the vast importance of condoms.

Condoms go a long way to preventing the spread of HIV, hepatitis B, C, D, etc., herpes, thrush, and various other irksome trifles you may find it hard to explain away.

Insist that if ever your O were to find him/herself in the unlikely position of cheating on you he/she'd ensure that condoms were used. If you find yourself in an unexpected/expected deceitful interlude, be sure, for the ongoing health of all concerned, that condoms are used.

Moreover, condoms have the added advantage of helping to prevent unwanted pregnancies, for which purpose they were coincidentally originally invented.

Many (misguided) modern lovers have a problem with condoms.

For some, it's the fear they'll appear contrived/premeditated for having one at the ready.

For some it's the fear of the sexual charge diminishing while they hunt for the packet, rip it open with their teeth, and fumble around with the condom, trying to put it on with one hand while maintaining the sexual link with the other. First putting it on the wrong way around so it only goes over the helmet (glans) then having to turn it around the other way. Then having to use both hands to stretch it out and pull it on over their now possibly wilting dick. And then back to, now where were we? I mean, how would James Bond do it?

But look, how often are your successful seductions (of short- or long-term Os) truly spontaneous, without premeditation or contrivance, to some degree at least? (Come on, admit it.)

So why be coy about it? Take the condom out before you even begin the whole sexual thing. Say, "Look, I have this!" and say it proudly and with conviction. What, you shouldn't want to have sex, or something? Who're you kidding? Everybody wants it. And everybody knows that. So don't pretend. Don't put your hand in your pocket or in your bedside drawer surreptitiously and pull out a condom with an "Oh, look what I've found!" as if you were actually checking to see if you had your car keys.

Or just keep one discreetly handy, literally to hand, so you can take it between thumb and forefinger at the appropriate moment, after your/O's version of "Shall I put a condom on now?" or "I want to feel you inside me—have you got a condom?"

Then stop what you're doing. And, sitting proudly back on your heels, thighs spread at a manly angle, using both hands, slowly, deliberately, open the wrapping, take the condom out, and make a zen/Tao meditative, integrated, unified action of putting it slowly and deliberately over your erect cock. Not shy. Not coy. But confidently and with conviction. (She'll love it. Confidence and conviction are *soooo* sexy.)

Make sure it's not split at the end, or likely to ride up and get lost inside, by stretching it fully over your dick. This part should be sexy for you, a bit like jerking off. At least that's the way to approach it.

A close friend of your author, too famous to mention, who once won a competition for condom application (her prize was a vibrator which the cat eventually chewed), also recommends that you hold the teat between thumb and forefinger of one hand while rolling the condom down over the penile shaft with the other. She was telling it from the vantage point of the woman, many of whom prefer to be the one to apply the prophylactic.

While moving your body in the coital dance, check every now

and then with one hand that the condom's rim is still around the base of the penis. While doing this, you may wish to take the opportunity to play around a bit with that hand or the fingers thereof. Someone's sure to enjoy that.

Eventually, after the last drop of semen has been squirted from your shuddering manhood and your willy begins to slowly deflate as the volume of blood diminishes, use your fingers to steady the rim of the condom against the base of your cock and slowly pull out/away, keeping hold of the condom's rim as you do. Perform this delicate operation, slowly but surely, well before the penis goes soft to avoid it slipping off inside and spilling its load in the wrong place at the wrong time.

When you're ready, boys can use a tissue, or bare hands if tissues or paper towels are not available, to carefully remove the by now floppy jellyfish-like prophylactic from the tip and dispose of it in a convenient garbage can.

And I nearly forgot. Another reason people (boys) find condoms irksome is the penile desensitizing factor, i.e., you don't feel so acutely through your dick. This, however, can be useful in reducing the effects of excess penile excitation that often lead (quickly) to sudden, unexpected ejaculation. Moreover, the penile desensitizing effect is largely offset by following the following.

Turning your whole body into an erogenous zone

There is a common misconception about erogenous zones, namely that there are certain points on the body which, when stimulated/teased, produce an erotic effect.

While it's true that each individual has points on the body which are more sensitive than others, more linked energically or by unconscious association to sexual/sensual pleasure stimulation, it's actually not so much the point you stimulate, but the *way* you stimulate it that will determine how much turn-on factor you generate.

Rather than focusing all your pleasure-giving attention to O's *genito-nippular* axis, i.e., nipples–clitoris/penis, spread your attention around their entire physical (and psychic) being. Kiss the earlobe of the ear that usually spends its time listening to people's voices on the phone. Suck the toe of the foot that usually stands within a shoe on the floor of Congress. Lick the forearm of the arm that usually holds up the hand whose finger points at the defendant in the courtroom. Let your nipple caress the shin that supports the knee that usually rises to deliver a front-kick. Transport each body part away from its usual workaday routine and into the erotic arena.

Every part of O's body is potentially erotically charged to varying degrees. Break out of the regular old nipples, clitoris/penis, earlobes, side of neck, back of neck, and anus routine. Imagine O's whole body is a giant erogenous zone.

When conditions, energy, and inclination permit, take time to discover the high points and low points of O's erotic/erogenous response, explore the peaks and valleys. Spend time in the valley before ascending to the peak. Give the event dynamics, i.e., rise and fall/light and shade/Yin and Yang. You can't hang out on the peak all night/day, it's too windy.

As the recipient O, visualize your entire body as a huge penis/clitoris. Don't be too hungry for genital stimulation. Enjoy being explored and played with all over (up and down the length of the land).

Feigning/exaggerating pleasure/faking an orgasm

Why do we all do this (from time to time)?

To make something special out of something dull.

Because we're so used to playing our part in the daily round of living theater that we don't know how to stop, and just feel.

Because we want to make Os feel good about themselves. (So we can hang on to them, perhaps.)

Because we want to give Os the impression that we're fully realized, flowing, unblocked sexual beings.

Because we don't wish to appear sexually inadequate/malfunctioning.

Because we like the sound of our own grunts/groans/moans/cries/screams/giggles.

You tell me.

As for faking orgasms, this practice is widespread to the point of ubiquity. And not just with the girls. Boys do it too. Not the ejaculation, but the moaning, groaning, and grunting that goes with it is often added to increase dramatic effect.

And why not? It's fun to act. It also provides a surefire way to end a liaison swiftly and effectively, when you can't think of a more elegant way to do it. Simply tell O you've been faking all along.

However, faking, as you know, isn't a patch on the real thing, and for the sake of your upcoming explorations into the labyrinthine world of Taoist sexology, it is rather important that you *Stop faking, stop acting,* and *drop the pretense* immediately, in order that you may instead devote all your sexual attention to feeling what you're actually feeling as you feel it.

More on the importance of physical fitness, flexibility, suppleness, and stamina

Though the practice of Taoist sex does not necessitate acts of gross contortionism or great feats of athletic prowess, and does in fact stress the need to develop softness (except for the obvious exception) during sex, it is important that your body is fit, flexible, supple, and strong enough to move in and out of any position you (and O) choose, without needing to visit a chiropractor immediately after the session.

A protracted session, as often tends to occur when using the Taoist approach, requires great stamina. The positions you find yourself in require flexibility of neck and hips (at least). The thrust and pump require solid strength in hips and lower back, and the ability to wriggle gracefully between positions requires suppleness.

Moreover, it is far more pleasing to most Os you'll encounter to grab hold of a form that feels alive, active, and toned, rather than some flabby, flaccid pile of untrained flesh. (Don't you think?)

To which end, it is recommended that you allocate/dedicate a regular portion of every day to attending to the fitness, flexibility, suppleness, and stamina levels of your physical person by means of intelligently performed daily physical exercise.

A fully rounded regime would include yoga/power-yoga/kundalini-yoga for flexibility, tai chi/martial arts for suppleness and grace, push-ups, sit-ups, free-weights and general gym activity for fitness and strength, and running/cycling/walking for stamina.

The younger you start, the better, but it's never too late. Begin now, by putting down the very handbook you are now reading and doing some of the above. (See you soon.)

Even if it's just for vanity's sake, start and maintain a regime of intelligent daily exercise comprised of your own version of the above, not just to enhance your sex, but to enhance everything you do (from now on).

It's much easier to feel sexy as you enter the sexual arena when you don't feel like you have to hold your stomach in, clench your buttocks, or strain to make your shoulders look broader, i.e., when you feel relatively confident about the visual gift you're bringing O's way.

Intensification
of sexual tension

When it is evident to both you and O that levels of sexual tension between you are running high, do not rush to reduce them by having sex with each other.

As a Taoist experiment, where/when applicable, spend up to three weeks or more letting levels intensify. Give yourself time to appreciate O fully before going through the sexual intimacy barrier together.

This can be effectively achieved by initially only spending up to half an hour together at any one time. Not long enough to ever have to have an argument or severely get on one another's nerves. Then, when you eventually spend four hours in bed together, the charge built up will be something worth releasing. However, there is also the danger of disappointment, which is why you must resist going into expectation mode about it. Simply tease without guile or expectation.

You must also be sensitive to the right moment at which to stop the tease and get on with the main event, as excess teasing/stimulation eventually deadens response.

Breathing

Breathing is obviously fairly important in a general sort of way, as not doing it for too long leads quite instantaneously to the demise of your person as you know it. Ask anyone into self-strangulation who went on just that little bit too long.

On a less melodramatic level, forgetting to breathe freely, especially in stressful and/or exciting situations, sky-diving, and/or sex, for example, generates even more stress/excitement, which puts a severe strain on your system, impairing your ability to do what has to be done and enjoy it. In extreme cases, it overloads your system, your heart packs up, and you end up just the same as if you went for the total breath-retention option above.

Breathe in fully. Breathe out fully. And don't hold your breath on the way out. Keep your diaphragm moving up and down. When you breathe in, let your belly expand. When you breathe out, let your belly contract. Let your chest remain relatively still/stable throughout.

But you don't have to make a fuss about it. No big breathing noises. No sitting up straight like a new-age goody-two-shoes and making big breathing motions. No stopping whatever you're doing, and with a spiritual poker face, making a big deal about it.

Just breathe. Quietly. Naturally. Like a baby. *Without* holding your breath.

Slowing the breath tempo

Do this to slow the tempo of your mind.

Do *that* to slow down the action.

Why would you want to slow down the action?

According to Taoists, Wayward *and* Traditional, as well as other assorted yogis, sorcerers, shamans, and general mountebanks, you only have a finite amount of breaths allocated to you in any one lifetime. So you might as well breathe slowly if you want the action to last longer.

This doesn't make it any less satisfying. To the contrary, it affords you the time to register, assimilate, savor, and appreciate the action as it's happening.

Far more satisfying than hurtling headlong down the track like the Orange Blossom Special, so fast you don't quite notice what's going on around you.

You don't quite notice how truly magnificent it is to be here in O's arms, your limbs entwined, your tongues teasing each other, your eyes gazing lovingly. You don't quite notice what a miracle that is. Because you're breathing too quickly.

Breathe slowly. Especially if you're a boy and you feel yourself starting to climb the slope of no return and it's clearly too soon. Slow your breath down, breathe deeply, fully, gently, and silently, and your runaway excitement will be brought back under control.

Breathing together
(with O)

There will be times, maybe even later on tonight, who knows, when you will be called upon by this author to attempt various techniques with O, of a meditative/inner-alchemical nature.

In some you will be breathing in as O is breathing out, in a Yin-Yang kinda way.

In others you will be breathing in as O is breathing in and breathing out as O is breathing out, in a Yang-Yang-Yin-Yin kinda way.

In yet others you will be asked to consciously retain (hold) your breath, as in a lungful, together. [See *The Big Squeeze*, p. 117.]

Of course, there will be times while engaged in sexual union with O, when you find it expedient/appropriate to practice your inner-alchemical chops on your own, totally unbeknown to O. In these instances, simply synchronize your breathing with O's.

Don't do too much with it. Just be aware of whether you're doing the Yin-Yang or the Yin-Yin-Yang-Yang.

At the most basic level, being in tune consciously with your breath at all times is enough to maintain a meditative state of conscious awareness (at all times). Especially when you're having sex.

Fancy postures

There are many fancy sexual postures in our universe, some of which are known to humans, a few of which are even in this book.

However, it's not the posture so much as the consciousness/love you express through it.

The most important thing is that both you and O are fully comfortable in your bodies. For this purpose it can be useful to always carry a stack of scatter cushions around with you, or if this proves impractical, to keep them near or on your bed/floor/kitchen table, etc. Use them judiciously to prop up body parts that would otherwise be straining against gravity, in order to reduce all excess/extraneous strain from the musculoskeletal systems of both you and O.

The postures presented herewith are all easy to get into and maintain, but are obviously more so the more fit, flexible, supple, and strong you are. The only guideline is not to attempt a posture that pushes your physical capabilities beyond where you've taken them before, unless you're willing to risk injury in your quest to fulfill your potential in this life. [See *Warning and disclaimer*, p. 3.]

If you find yourself in an awkward position and your lower back hurts, the circulation in your left arm is being cut off, you think your neck might snap or your tongue lock, don't be shy about negotiating a quick transformation of the physical configuration, i.e., move, you twit.

As soon as you feel uncomfortable in any position, doing no matter what, rearrange yourself/yourselves until you don't. Whichever stage of the proceedings you are at, even if O's just about to come, if you feel pain in your back, chest, joints, or you think you might pass out for lack of air, move.

There are no awards for people who martyr themselves in the Coliseum of Sexual Love (my friend).

Relaxation

Didn't your mom ever tell you? If you want to come (properly), relax your hips.

Conversely, if you don't want to come (properly), relax your hips.

In short, relaxing your hips helps you do everything properly.

However, it would be unfair to many other fine body parts if your hips were to take all the credit. In fact, it's true to say that if you want to have truly rude and amazing (love and) sex, relax your entire body.

In fact, it's even true to say that if you want to have a truly amazing *life*, relax your entire body.

But as any good urban warrior knows, relaxing does not mean collapsing. Relaxing means consciously using only as much physical strength as is necessary to do what you have to do and no more. If it is necessary for you to tense your thighs momentarily to enable you to thrust your hips forward, for example, why do you also tense the back of your neck? It's unnecessary. Stop it. Relax.

Relaxation means allowing the natural Yin-Yang dynamic of hold and release that occurs of itself as you do the sexual dance, without adding any unnecessary tension to the proceedings.

Don't use sex as a way of releasing your tension. All you'll do is transmit tension to O, who'll transmit it back to you. Tension Ping-Pong.

Relax before (and during) sex.

If you think this vital piece of information might be difficult for you to later implement in real-time, say and/or write this affirmation about eighty-one times:

I relax when I'm having sex.

Hell, relax anyway, dude.

Four ounces

Whatever you do in the sexual dance, apply no more than four ounces of pressure.

Do you mean I have to carry my pocket scales at all times?

No. You can sense four ounces.

How?

Well, three ounces is too light/insipid for your touch to transmit and receive sexual love, and five ounces is too heavy/intrusive and will block the flow/mutual interchange.

Four ounces is a metaphor. It's another way of saying touch with love, respect, sensitivity, and wonder at the miracle of O's presence at such close range, and with appreciation of that miracle.

It's like eating a gourmet meal. A gastronomically sophisticated diner is sensitive/sensuous enough to take the time to savor the delicate taste-combinations released in each mouthful, enjoying the physical sensation of chewing and relaxing thoracically to allow the food to slip down easily into the stomach. This is all done with respect and appreciation for the time, energy, and expertise of the chef, as well as all the other people involved in the chain of hunting, gathering, cultivating, distributing, delivering, preparing, and serving the meal. Eventually, napkin is raised to delicately dab the lips, a discreet burp escapes into its laundered folds, and gourmet sits back to contemplate the selection of cheeses.

That's a four-ounce approach.

Now picture an uncouth, unwashed, smelly, overweight, ugly, hairy, hungry, ornery, foul-mouthed ogre/ogress preparing to eat the same meal. About to woof it back like an industrial vacuum cleaner and gobble it down like a hungry beast, he/she notices that the meal's not actually there because it's just been eaten by the gourmet. So he/she whacks the gourmet so hard, his face lands in the Stilton.

That is not the four-ounce approach.

It's not so different with sex.

Keep your whole body active and sensitive. Never let part or all of your body be slumped on O's body like a lump of dead meat.

Maintain contact pressure at a steady four-ounce at all times, whether touching, stroking, kissing, licking, sucking, fucking, or simply frolicking.

The Big Squeeze

To facilitate the orgasmic state of sexual nirvana, it is essential to get a grip (pun) on the Big Squeeze. This is a modern Wayward Taoist term for a very traditional/ancient Taoist technique.

It is entertaining to think of all the big squeezers that have gone before in the previous five or six millennia as you perform this technique.

It is employed at the precise moment that the preorgasmic charge has intensified to such a high level that you're either going to explode from the genitals or blow your head off. One nano-second before the very final point of no return.

So there you are, boy-O, faced with a split-second choice to make: go the way of the hedonist and explode from the genitals, or the way of the Wayward Taoist hedonist and blow your head off.

You've done a lot of the former in your time, some great, some not so great, and yes, the temptation's strong, but, no (you think), this time I'm going to try something a little different. Something a bit spiritual, to further me on my journey of self-development, something to launch me into the stratospheric heavenly orgasmic realm of sexual nirvana. I'm going to blow my fucking head off. (Metaphorically speaking.) [See *Warning and disclaimer*, p. 3.]

Your split-second choice is made. (You're going for the Big Squeeze.)

And this is what you do:

One: internally pull up (contract) your perineum.

My what?

The point directly behind your genitals and directly in front of your anus. That in-between bit. Taoists call it the Gate of Mortality.

Why?

Because if the sexual charge (chi stored in your sacral region) passes through the Gate and explodes through your genitals, it reaffirms your mortality, i.e., reconfirms your ticket on the wheel of life and death ride, as in sperm makes babies, babies grow up, you grow older, and then you die.

However, if the sexual charge (chi) does not pass through the Gate, you can send it up along your spinal column into your brain, where it momentarily blows all sense of local self away as you drift in the formless state of sexual nirvana, beyond the clutches of linear time, where you have always been and will always be (for ever and ever). That is, you are now your Spirit Body and hence immortal.

Immortal? Isn't that overromanticizing things a bit?

Maybe. So what? Try it out for yourself and see.

Anyhow, you pull up the perineum as hard as you can, without creating any unnecessary (excess) muscular tension in the surrounding musculature, in order to lock the Gate of Mortality (so the sexual charge can't escape).

As you do so, start to squeeze the sexual charge (chi) inch by inch, higher and higher up your spine. To enable the sexual charge (chi) to reach all the way up into your brain (upper TT), relax and lengthen the back of your neck, push your tongue hard up against the roof of your mouth, and roll your eyes up (behind your eyelids) to gaze "heavenward."

Take a deep breath in to the count of nine and hold it (without straining) for nine counts (at your natural counting tempo).

Maintain the squeeze. Release the breath gently to the count of nine.

Breathe in again to the count of nine, and so on, repeating the in for nine, hold for nine, release for nine pattern, up to nine times, all the while maintaining the perineal squeeze, the relaxed, lengthened neck, the pushed-up tongue, and the rolled-back eyes (without straining), and feel the charge blow your head off (into sexual nirvana land).

After nine breath cycles, or whenever you've had enough, roll your eyes gently back into position, drop your tongue back into resting position on your lower palate, and slowly release your perineum, allowing the chi to slowly drop down the front of your spine into your lower TT (below the navel).

The benefits traditionally associated with this practice include spiritual immortality, spiritual enlightenment, evolved psychic/clairvoyant powers, strengthened endocrine/immune system, increased vitality, bright eyes, and the ability to maintain erections without surprise, unwanted ejaculation, for as long as you choose.

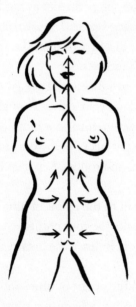

If both you and O do the Big Squeeze simultaneously, you may experience complete psychospiritual bonding, unlike any other kind of bonding you may have hitherto experienced. You may find yourselves with complete empathetic telepathy, unbounded by physical form, floating free together in an infinite ocean of sexual love, like two halves of the Buddha, the archetypal Yin and Yang of the Great Tao itself.

Then again, you may not. Either way, it behooves you to train yourself by practicing the Big Squeeze on your own as an internal callisthenics interlude, on a daily basis, until you are completely comfortable/confident with the sequence, before trying it out with O.

Build up strength in your perineum by doing eighty-one light, quick-action squeeze-and-releases every day (Squeeze Lite). This is important as it helps prevent aching-balls-the-next-day syndrome, which can occur from incorrect sperm-retention practice during sex.

When rolling your eyes upward, be sure not to use force or you risk detaching your retina. [See *Warning and disclaimer*, p. 3.]

When training yourself in the Big Squeeze, it is helpful sometimes, when in the mood, to practice while masturbating (obviously).

If I was restricted to teaching/sharing only one technique in this whole handbook, the Big Squeeze would be the one. (That's how much we love it.)

The question of orgasms

There is no question. Orgasms are one of the most important things in life. Do you realize the crazy things people get up to in order to have one?

However, the point (if there actually is one) in practicing Wayward Taoist sex is not to achieve or help O achieve an orgasm. Orgasms are not the point. Even heavenly spiritual orgasms are not the point.

The point is merely to be present. Be present with O whatever. Whether you come and/or O comes or not. The orgasm is not the goal. If there is a goal, it is to share something of authentic beauty from your heart and soul with O and receive the same back.

The orgasm if/when it happens is merely part of that process. A nice part. But just a part.

You are not responsible for giving O an orgasm.

O is not responsible for giving you one.

Each individual carries full responsibility for his/her own orgasm.

If you know the only way you're going to come properly is to manually or otherwise stimulate your own clitoris, or have O do it for you, while he's inside you, then it's your responsibility to communicate your needs/wants as they arise and to position yourself accordingly, if you are intent on having an orgasm.

If you (O-girl) like to orgasm once, twice, or more before boy-O does, it's your responsibility to somehow communicate this clearly.

Ideally, boy-O is so self-attuned that he intuits your needs/wants and organizes fulfilling his own around them. But this is not always the case. Just as it is not always the case (boy-O) that an O-girl will intuit yours.

To this end, it is well that you do the following.

Use your voice (to talk/moan) during sex

Always be proud to vocalize; do not be ashamed/embarrassed/shy of passing air along your vocal cords in order to produce sound, in either formal linguistic style, i.e., words, phrases, or sentences, or freestyle, i.e., moans, groans, squeals, giggles, grunts, ohs, oos, ahs, and/or various combinations thereof, in order to communicate your pleasure/displeasure, appreciation, wants and needs, and/or to arrange a mutually convenient moment to come together.

And of course it's OK to assume a "sexy" vocal tone/timbre and indeed give expression to your complete vocal range during sex.

And it's OK to use silly words, terms of endearment, "dirty" talk, and blatant euphemisms to disguise your discomfort/embarrassment.

Hell, it's even OK to do baby talk, if you really must.

But it's *so* much sexier to be yourself. Be natural. Sure, talk quietly so you don't deafen O, but talk like you normally do. Enunciate your words properly. Speak in plain sentences. Don't try to use "sexy" words. Be yourself.

If you feel embarrassed, just remember embarrassment is the closest thing to bliss. Be embarrassed, it doesn't matter. Say what you want to say, as you want to say it, when you want to say it. You only look stupid when you're embarrassed about being embarrassed. If you're not embarrassed about being embarrassed, it just looks sexy when you talk through the embarrassment.

This doesn't mean that you should purposely render your speech coarse or in any way irksome to the ear, just to prove you're "being" natural. Just *be* natural.

Don't exaggerate your desire to moan, groan, or grunt because you think it makes you look more uninhibited/wild/exciting as a lover. Neither should you suppress sound that wants to come out in case it reveals too much of your animal/bestial self.

(Obviously there will be times when you find it expedient to control the output level so as not to disturb uninvolved others in the vicinity.)

Remember that the sound quality of your voice is more important than the content of your words. Use your voice to sonically massage O's ears/brain/consciousness. Do this by relaxing your throat and thorax, rather than by trying to sound sexy.

Let any sound you make rise up from between your legs, so that it carries your sexual energy in its vibrations. That's what makes it sound sexy.

When using the spoken word to communicate your desires, do so clearly, confidently, and with conviction, because that's sexy. Don't be afraid that talking will break the sexual spell. If that should occur, relax and just enjoy the conversation. The sex will come around again later. Say what you say under the umbrella of the sexual spell. In other words, don't break the sexual connection just because you're talking.

Above all, when intending to communicate a desire to O, do not mumble or swallow your words out of embarrassment, thus causing O to keep asking, "What? Pardon? What did you say?"

If, however, you find yourself on the receiving end of an embarrassed mumble, don't let the "What? Pardon? What did you say?" thing break the spell. Ask it as many times as you need to find out what the devil O wants *this* time.

Inner alchemy

This is a grandiose way of describing the process whereby you cause chi to circulate around specific psychic pathways in your body/Spirit Body, using your breath and mental focus, in order to transmute sexual chi in your lower Tan Tien (belly/loins) into refined cosmic chi, i.e., sexual nirvana fuel, in your upper Tan Tien (center brain/Ni Wan Peaks), in order to become a fully realized being (or just so you can tell people at parties that that's what you do so they think you're really cool).

It is helpful, before trying this with O, to train solo for a while in the following method, known to urban warriors as "Scoopin' the Loop," as it forms the basis of "Whooshing the Chi," which is what you do with O when you've got the sexual nirvana thing going—when you find yourselves intertwined in the highest realms of sexual-love consciousness and are wondering what to do next.

Scoopin' the Loop is simple.

Running up the back of your spine from between your legs to the top of your head and down behind the front of your skull to the roof of your mouth, is an invisible/psychic energy channel/tube.

Running from your lower palate, down the front of your spinal column, behind your pubic bone to your perineum, is another invisible/psychic energy channel/tube.

The back channel carries Yin energy upward so it becomes Yang. The front channel carries Yang energy downward so it becomes Yin.

When you push your tongue up onto the roof of your mouth, you form what's known in the trade as the "magpie bridge," which forms a connection between the two channels.

This facilitates an uninterrupted circular flow of energy which Yin-Yangs both your physical body and Spirit Body into some semblance of order. This order is crucial for both your physical health, and your psychic stability, and is necessary to prevent your becoming spiritually disheveled, disorientated, and/or distorted by the fierce altered states sometimes engendered by Taoist practices, especially the sexual variety. Moreover, being properly Yin-Yanged provides you with a natural force field to protect you from harmful acts of energy vampirism and psychic-draining performed wittingly or otherwise by Os with a negative energy charge. (This happens more frequently than you might imagine.)

Once you can visualize/feel these channels, the next stage is to let your mind slowly track the circuit, starting at your perineum, ascending the back channel, climbing over the brain, down to the upper palate, through the magpie bridge, and down the front channel to the perineum again.

As you get used to tracking the circuit with your mind, begin to introduce breathing awareness. At first, breathe in and out as if you're operating a hydraulic pump which pushes your mind around the circuit.

When you feel more confident, simply breathe in to push energy up the back channel and down into the roof of your mouth; breathe out to push the mind down through the magpie bridge along the front channel and into the perineum again.

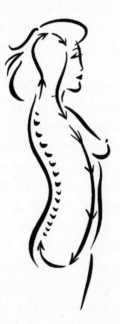

The blend of breath awareness and moving mind in turn pushes the chi around the loop.

Scoop nine good loops a day and major magic will come your way. (*Olé.*)

If you are interested in practicing this inner alchemy in tandem with an O, i.e., Whooshing the Chi, thus doing the kind of psychosexual bonding that takes you to extreme places, it is essential for you to Scoop the Loop alone every day.

[See *Whoosing the Chi*, p. 199.]

Cold sex vs. warm sex

Always care about the person you're having sex with, whether it's someone you've known intimately for an hour or a lifetime.

If you don't care about the person, and I don't mean the physical appearance, but the heart and soul of that person, if you don't empathize with their existential pain as well as their pleasure, the sex will be cold.

Cold sex is like acting out a pornographic movie in order to satisfy some secret fucked-up agenda of your own. It ices your heart over and is detrimental to your psychic health, pokes holes in your aura, weakens your immune system, and is generally depleting for all parties concerned. Otherwise it's fine.

Warm sex arises simply from caring about O. Just as you'd care for your own child. It's a bit like being a parent and lover at the same time. This should not be mistaken, however, for over-caring, which is a disguised manipulative control device.

If you truly care about yourself, let your sex be warm.

Visualize a jet of crimson-gold-colored light streaming from the middle of your chest (middle Tan Tien) and enveloping O with love. Do this in your imagination and while actually having sex with O in real-time.

Planning the moment vs. letting the moment happen

In reality, it's usually a combination of both. You set the context, create the environment, have a shower, have condoms ready (if appropriate), and have everything sorted so that if the energy moves you both that way, you end up having sex that night/ day/whatever.

You can't force, coerce, manipulate, threaten, or cajole O into sharing sexual love with you. Sex maybe, but not sexual love.

You can't force Eros to present himself. You can but create the context/space and allow the Tao to do the rest.

The Tao of the situation can be affected, however, by Wu Wei. Wu Wei means getting something you want (if it's what's healthiest for everyone involved and in accordance with the free will of everyone involved) without any effort on your part whatsoever, just by intending a desired outcome.

O's coming over tonight and you really want to fuck him/her. So you say to the Tao, as in your own higher, universal self, "I really want to fuck O tonight if it's in accordance with the Tao of the situation." Then you get in touch with the feeling you want to feel as a result of having made love with O. Warm, loved, cherished, seen, known, cared for, and at one with yourself, O, and all creation. Conjure the feeling as if the love/making has already happened. This sets up a suitable resonance for O to respond to, if O should choose.

Then let the whole thing go. Just give it to the Tao of the situation to take care of for you.

When O comes around, it turns out it doesn't matter to you

whether you make love or not because you already feel complete in yourself anyway.

This makes you far more approachable and desirable on an energic level.

So you win either way.

In other words, plan the moment, then let it happen on its own.

Acting out fantasies

It's fun to act out your fantasies about O with O in real-time. As long as O is willing. For this to happen you need to communicate your desire to act out your fantasy and gain O's consent before proceeding to act it out. Otherwise you're acting it out at O's expense.

It's fine to indulge in playing charades as long as all the players know that's what's happening.

Moreover, telling O your fantasy ahead of time can be so damn sexy you may well end up acting out stuff spontaneously, as a result, that surpasses your fantasy by twenty-three leagues (or more).

The question
of masturbation

It hasn't been that long since masturbation was generally considered a heinous crime against nature, frequent indulgence in which would lead swiftly to blindness, insanity, and eventually death.

While I've heard of one young man, who'd taken Viagra and vitamin E, jerking himself off so hard, long, and furiously in the toilets at a club that he actually rubbed the skin off his dick and required surgery and a skin graft, I've never heard of anyone actually jerking himself to death. Interesting way to go though, I suppose, wondering if this is the one that's going to kill you just before you come each time.

Fact is, everybody jerks off at some time or other (at least).

People do it to get to sleep.

People do it for comfort, as a distraction, because they feel horny and don't know how to get themselves laid that day, because they've got a fantasy about someone they want to explore alone, because they find themselves irresistibly attractive, or simply because they're wankers. So what?

It's no big deal that people piss, shit, sneeze, vomit, eat, fart, sit, stand, walk, run, or jump up and down on the spot, so why is it a big deal if they jerk off? It's just a natural function.

Obviously, if you're so into it that you can't get on with your life, you'll have to go to WA (Wankers Anonymous). Otherwise, carry on as you were. Just be sure to wipe up properly after yourself (where appropriate).

Some Os, maybe even you yourself, enjoy jerking themselves off in each other's company, which can provide many fine minutes of fun, especially when maintaining eye contact. However, if you find this becoming habitual and forming a pattern, you might consider exploring your issues of boundaries, control, and intimacy with an experienced therapist.

Some men like to jerk off before going out on a hot date, so that they won't get too horny and blow the seduction or come too soon. However, practicing the Big Squeeze is recommended as a less sticky alternative.

Masturbation is more or less essential if you want to get to know/reacquaint yourself with your own sexuality. Once you do, however, you might consider saving the energy for your next time with O.

The question of sperm retention

There has been much heavyweight bullshit propagated over the years about the Taoist concept of sperm retention.

The true Taoist attitude to sperm retention, as it is with all things, is that if it arises of itself, fine. If you're forcing it, it'll eventually make you ill.

By practicing the Big Squeeze both every day as a solo exercise and when having sex with O, as well as Scoopin' the Loop on a regular basis, you may well find the need to ejaculate diminishes of itself.

Every time a man ejaculates he uses up a portion of jing or "ancestral chi." This is a particular kind of energy inherited from your ancestral line at conception, equivalent to the idea of DNA. You inherit a finite amount of jing. When it's all used up you die. So obviously, the less often you ejaculate, the less you accelerate your demise.

However, this does *not* mean you should never ejaculate, or that you should ejaculate only when you want to conceive a baby. That would be like having a fortune in the bank but living in poverty and squalor.

In fact, providing you're fairly healthy and your kidneys, which store the jing, are kept in reasonably good shape, the odd squirt and shudder from time to time won't make that much difference to your longevity.

Men in their mid-forties (like me) are advised to reduce the frequency of ejaculation during winter months as the cold weather adversely affects the kidneys. But to put an arbitrary figure on how many times a week/month/year you're safe to ejaculate without risking your longevity is entirely idiotic as everyone's constitution is different.

It's more important *how* you ejaculate than how often.

If your ejaculation is strong, unfettered by inhibition, guilt, and/or shame, and the cause of your ejaculation has been a session of good loving sex with a loving, caring O, that will do you more good than sitting in the corner on your own, like a sperm miser clutching on to your balls.

When going for sexual nirvana, it's perfectly viable to sustain the state of perpetual heavenly orgasmic bliss for as long as you feel like it, and then reverse the flow, release the perineal lock, open the Gate of Mortality, and ejaculate to your scrotum's content if you should so choose. But if you decide not to go for the ejaculation option and retain the sperm instead, you may find you can sustain the nirvanic state for longer, leaving you feeling energized and invigorated.

Either way, it's the nirvanic state that makes you enlightened, not holding on to your sperm.

Far more important that you learn how to enjoy a full, unbridled, uninhibited, orgasmic ejaculation, without any negative postorgasmic slapback, and get used to that so it becomes ordinary to you, before you let go completely and forget about ejaculating altogether.

Women, on the other hand, are encouraged to come as often and as much as they want, as it actually builds their jing. (Lucky things.)

Dirty, what's dirty?

Providing that all body parts including orifices of all parties concerned, as well as all surfaces that may be used to support part or all of any body involved in the action, and providing that all parties desist from urinating, defecating, vomiting, or otherwise sullying themselves or each other during sexual proceedings, there's nothing *dirty* about sex. Nothing dirty at all.

When people talk about dirty sex, they either mean uninhibited, i.e., natural, healthy sex, or they mean sticking your finger, tongue, or penis into someone's asshole, the dirtiness factor of which depends on the cleanliness of all fingers, tongues, dicks, and assholes involved.

Eyes open vs. eyes closed

It's beautiful to watch O in the throes of ecstasy.

So don't feel obliged to close your eyes because you think it might be considered impolite to stare. Keep your eyes open if you want and watch the show (it's riveting).

Moreover, and more important, gazing into the eyes of O while engaged in coitus, and allowing O to gaze into yours, exponentially deepens the soul connection between you.

Stare into each other's eyes from a distance of twenty-six inches or so, while not having sex, without looking away, until your peripheral vision dissolves, and O's face dissolves and starts to transform itself into different versions of O's face, revealing (some say) the faces of all O's past lives; revealing (others say) all the archetypes including the devil; and ultimately revealing O's Original Face (before O was born), i.e., the divine nature of O. Maintain your mutual gaze for up to six minutes or more, or until one or the other of you gets bored with it. Then try it the next time you're having sex together (if you want).

Conversely, it is equally important, especially when engaged in the Big Squeeze, Whooshing the Chi, and drifting in sexual nirvana, to close your eyes and lose yourself in the experience.

Sometimes you keep your eyes open to maintain control over the situation, in case, for example, O should suddenly pull a gun on you and steal your money, drugs, or whatever. Except in certain extreme cases, this will usually prove to be somewhat overvigilant, however, so if you find yourself doing this, experiment with closing your eyelids for a while and losing control.

Sometimes you may find yourself locking your eyes shut because consciously or unconsciously, you/part of you don't/doesn't really want to be there. If you find yourself doing this, experiment with sneaking a quick peek at the action every now and then and see how it makes you feel. If it turns out you don't really want to be there, go. [See *You're free to do whatever you choose*, p. 34.]

Stopping when you want

You are always free (and this must be clearly understood and appreciated by both you and O) to stop at any time in the proceedings. Even if it's just before O's about to come, if you want to stop, stop.

It's perfectly OK for you to kiss, suck, tease, stroke, and then stop and leave both you and O hanging in midair, if you feel like it.

Kissing does *not* have to lead to foreplay. Foreplay does *not* have to end in fucking. Fucking does *not* have to end in coming. And coming does *not* have to end in lolling around in bed together for an hour or more talking nonsense to each other.

There is no set sequence to follow. There is no time limit on your sexual expression, save for any you and/or O place on it. You may suddenly enter O from behind without warning one morning when she's naturally wet and ready, for example, tease her with a few gentle thrusts, pull out without getting anywhere near to coming, then go and have a pee and a shower. Later, you may suddenly, with no malice aforethought, take her right nipple in your mouth and suck it for eight minutes or more, without uttering a single word of explanation or justification, then just as suddenly stop and go back to your breakfast.

Later still, you may, just out of the blue, take O in your arms and French-kiss her till you're both bursting out of your respective skins and then stop and go back to reading the paper.

A short while after that, O may grab you by the scruff of your neck and demand angrily, "Fuck me or get out!"

On the other hand, she may appreciate the tease and be able to contain her sexual energy enough to enjoy waiting for whatever comes next, whether it comes in a minute, an hour, a day, a month, or even a year from now (no rush).

It's perfectly fine to do little trailers or short films when you feel like it, without feeling obliged (to yourself or O) to follow up with the full-length feature every time.

A creative sex session can be spread out over a period of days, slowly building and intensifying the sexual tension between you until it reaches untenable proportions, and then having the fuck of your lives.

It doesn't all have to be done, wiped up, and got out of the way in an hour and three minutes.

Just as a serious chess match can be played over a period of weeks, even months, and as a fine banquet can be savored one course at a time over a period of many hours, so can one fuck be stretched out over a period of days if you've got the patience and inclination, and feel free, on either side, to stop immediately, whatever the action occurring at that instant, without fearing that you're offending O in any way.

Of course, you may also need to stop because you don't want to be there right now/ever again. You may suddenly realize you don't like O at all anymore. It happens.

And in that moment of limbo, while you choose whether to stop or continue . . . ah, now there's the bit you discuss with your therapist.

Stopping is also useful during the initial wooing stage of a situation, to prevent the action from racing ahead before the sexual tension has had a chance to build to optimum levels, i.e., the chemistry's had time to settle into a workable compound.

Not that you should never sleep with someone on the first night. We don't live in a world of shoulds. If the energy leads you both to fuck within hours/minutes/seconds of first meeting each other, then that's where you go (in reality). It's just that because you don't really know each other (at all), you may (both) find it uncomfortable or awkward after all that sudden intimacy, trying to make postorgasmic conversation, as in "What's your name?" etc. Then again, you may not.

Stopping the internal commentary

What internal commentary?

You know: Wow, look at me now. If they could see me now (Wish they could/Glad they can't). Wow, she's so beautiful/Hum, she's not as beautiful as I thought she was. I wish he was Dan/Theo/Clancy instead. Oh, I shouldn't have thought that.

Umm, that's nice, I wish he'd do it again. Shall I say something? His elbow's digging into my upper arm and burning the skin. Shall I move my arm? Better not, it might put him off. Oh, God, I hope I'm not going to come now, I'm not even inside her yet. I bet Roger/Tarquin/Ojas the Hero would be able to hold it longer than this. Why can't I be a real man like them? Can she hear me thinking this? I wonder if my dick's big enough for her. I bet the last guy she was with had a bigger/smaller willy than I do. I wish I had a bigger/smaller dick. I can't feel anything/It's hurting—it feels like it's splitting me in two. I wonder if I want this relationship. How can I make her/him stay. Does she expect me to stay the night? What excuse can I make to get out of here after (and get back to my wife/husband/computer/own bed). God, I think I love her/him more than the universe. Shit, I don't think I love him/her anymore. How am I going to get out of this? Fuck, did I remember to phone Max? I wonder when he's/she's going to come. My God, this is the best sex I've/we've ever had. So what? God, how could I think "so what" about sex like this? Because it's only sex. And so on and so on. Round and round it goes. Chatter chatter. And everyone (at least, occasionally) falls prey to it. It's like driving the car, talking on the phone, and turning on the radio at the same time. It's easy to do.

The point, however, if you wish to plumb the Taoist sexual depths, is to stop the chatter. Get out of your head and into your body for as much time as you can during the session. (This applies to life in general, not just to sex specifically.)

The way to do this, as with any other style of meditation, is to first observe yourself going through the commentary. Simply be aware of it, without judging it as wrong or trying in any way to stop or override it. Be aware and breathe. Also be aware of your hips. Be aware of your chest. Be aware of the space behind your eyes. In short, be aware of your body. And as you breathe, simply allow the commentator to carry on, while you enjoy the sensations in your body. Just as you're aware of the football commentator while you watch the game on TV, but your focus is all on the game.

You use the commentary to anchor yourself in the familiar, in order not to let go and lose yourself in the new.

Far better for your personal growth, not to mention the sex, to anchor yourself in your hips instead.

The techniques and you

The Taoist sexual techniques presented in the next section of the handbook are meant as a guide. It is not intended for you to act them out in sequential order, sticking to the "correct" number of repetitions, following instructions to the letter. That might prove to be robotic and stiff.

There is a danger, when presenting a scheme, of encouraging a mechanistic approach, which I wish to avoid at all costs. So be watchful for any mechanistic tendencies that may arise in your practice. Integrate any technique that takes your fancy in a fluid way. Allow it to integrate *itself* into your behavioral repertoire, if you wish.

You'll probably find that many of the techniques comprise actions and/or fantasies you've already experienced naturally.

Sex is not about technique, it's about feeling and sharing. It is my hope that these techniques provide you with new forms and/or new angles on old forms, through which to feel and share (much) more fully/freely.

Do not take any of this—sex/technique/yourself/life/barefoot doctors, etc.—too seriously. It will spoil all the fun.

The perfect fuck
(here goes.)

You find yourself in a state of uncontrollable mutual desire, with O in a secluded setting appointed with perfect lighting, sound, decor, reclining facilities, and ambient smells. Both of you have ample time to spare and have agreed verbally or otherwise to engage each other in an open-ended sexual interlude, with no preset agenda to act out.

O feels beautiful, sexy, desirable, confident, romantic, eager, uninhibited, natural, free, irresistible, and magnificent, and looks it too.

You feel beautiful, sexy, desirable, confident, romantic, eager, uninhibited, natural, free, irresistible, and magnificent, and look it too.

O smells perfect. So do you. O tastes delicious, so do you.

O sounds *sooo* good and sooo do you.

The chemistry between you has been mixed in heaven. The sexual tension has built to optimum intensity.

You undress each other in a haze of romantic frenzy, your eyes thrilling to the sight as respective garments and undergarments are removed/torn off one by one.

You fall into an embrace that feels like the embrace of eternity, tongues reaching deep into each other's hungry mouths; your hands thrilling to the touch of the side of O's thigh, O's neck, kissing O's neck, O gasping, almost coming from the sound, breast rubs eye, penis, stiff and pressing against belly, rolling, writhing, O's leg between your thighs, moaning, loving, devouring, caressing, O biting your shoulder, you kissing O's belly, sucking nipple, licking clitoris. Licking penis, the glans. Locked licking each other's genitals, perineum, tongues darting into assholes. No shame. No holding back. Sexual pleasure mounting so high your soul might burst. Penetration. Intense thrill of entry. Slowly, tenderly filling, being filled. Moving, slowly, sensitive to each other's every nuance. Perfect rhythm. Perfect pace. Every nerve ending activated. Every sensation amplified a thousand times. No awareness of commentary. And it feels so warm. So loving. So tender. Yet so erotic. Raunchy. Yet elegant. Graceful. Like a heavenly ballet danced in the primordial forest. Multiple orgasms. Erections that haven't even begun to think about ejaculating yet. No anxiety. No fears of suddenly, surprisingly, shuddering and squirting. Everything is completely under control yet completely spontaneous and natural. No thinking. Just feeling. And you're starting to feel the Chi Whooshing around your body and you enhance it with your mind because you've both mastered everything in this handbook at an earlier date, and you're changing positions, from behind, O on top. You on top. This way. That way. Without ever pulling out. Just contact. An endless, unbroken circle of contact. And your consciousness is moving to a new level. You both do a Big Squeeze, Whoosh the Chi, another Big Squeeze, you wait, one moment, and *bang* you're floating together in sexual nirvana. No longer two separate beings, but one being, one with All Being, the Tao, where you dissolve into undifferentiated, absolute bliss. You feel your body again. O feels it too. You start to move, move more powerfully, from deeper in your hips and you both know it's time for explosion. Penis, swollen to bursting, fills vagina, pumping so it bangs up inside the brain, faster, stronger, and now, now, now. Now! The Universal Tao explodes as you do, big-bang style, shudders, ejaculates, shudders some more, ejaculates more, and more until you can't imagine where it's all coming from, and finally comes to rest in the space between your two hearts, beating together as you do another dissolve, this time into the soft warmth

of tender love you both feel, the gratitude to life and full appreciation of the miracle of each other's existence.

And then O does a loud, smelly fart and blows it all (kidding).

So what?

It's true. You can be doing the perfect fuck scenario, even having
the most mind-buggering orgasm of your life, and your mind can
still be thinking, "So what?"

Which is because everything you do, everything you feel, everything you experience, no matter how profound or sublime, is
merely a trick of the light. It's all a grand illusion. All there really
is is the Big Phat Tao sitting in the middle of Nothing and Everything, playing with itself.

And at the deepest level, your mind knows that.

You might think "so what?" is a slightly churlish response to
something as stupendous as the greatest orgasm of your life, but I
say it shows attitude. And the Tao likes a bit of that.

It's important to have enough "so what?" factor about you to
prevent your gushing too much and getting mushy. (It's very hard
to make gushing and mushy sexy.) Be cool about it. It's only sex.

'Nuff seduction?

You want to go into the bedroom now?

(Come on then.)

THE**STING**
(what you actually do)

Reminder

Don't be mechanical. Don't be clinical. Don't be intellectual. Don't be obedient (to the instructions/number of repetitions/sequence of techniques). Don't be impatient. Don't be scared. Don't pretend. Don't fart in bed.

Do use a condom (when you know you should). Do be intuitive (and use the instructions to fire off your own innate sexual knowledge). Do be flowing and natural. Do be gentle, tender, loving, caring, and warm. Do be authentic. Do empty your bladder and bowels discreetly (when necessary) before you start, so you don't expend valuable energy preventing same.

(Thank you.)

The following "techniques" are not intended to be followed in sequence. The sexual dance is circular, intuitive, and spontaneous. Pick 'n' mix your steps at will.

Gateway to the Soul in the sole

Touch the sole of O's foot exactly midway between the toes and heel, and midway between instep and outstep, i.e., dead center of the sole. Use your fingertip to do this.

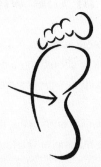

Maintain eye contact.

Move your finger in small circles eighteen times counterclockwise, eighteen times clockwise, massaging the flesh of the sole gently, as if undoing an ancient lock on an old treasure chest.

Touch one foot at a time or both together as the fancy takes you.

This is the Gateway to the Soul opening, which (by way of your finger-circling) gives you access to O's soul.

You might like to pause momentarily on completion to allow O's soul time to respond before continuing.

You might also like to invite O to open the Gateway to your Soul sometime.

Supporting the jade pillow

Place your palm at the back of O's neck where the neck meets the skull (occiput), so that your palm potentially provides a support for O's head. Allow O to give his/her head into your hand, i.e., trust, relax, and surrender. This provides comfort and makes O feel nurtured.

Maintain this hold for one minute twenty seconds, two frames and one bit, or until it feels like time to stop.

Wind in the willows

Position yourself comfortably with your slightly parted lips poised (without strain to your neck or shoulders) a centimeter above O's forearm, which is positioned so that your lips are able to brush the downy forearm hair at will.

Starting at the lower (wrist) end, lightly blow a line of air through the hair, blowing along the midline of O's forearm up to the upper (elbow) end, by moving your entire head along the forearm's length, thereby keeping the trajectory of expelled air perpendicular to its target.

When you've managed to work that out, remember this move requires a subtle motion of the hips to enable your spine to flex and bend easily. Be loose about it.

Between blows, breathe in deeply through your nose and allow the subtle smell of O's skin to wash up through your olfactory gates, straight to your reception desk.

Appreciate that this forearm is what connects O's soul to O's hand, and through that hand O interacts with the world. Through this forearm, you're connecting with O's life story, and as you know, that's sexy. (Though that might depend on the story.)

Repeat this up-and-down-the-forearm motion thrice, or there-abouts, and if you're enjoying it and O seems to indicate likewise, use your lips to caress the ends of the hairs as you blow.

Three slow runs up and down later, if you begin to notice a sexual charge building, allow your lips to kiss along the line, up and down thrice. You can then follow kissing with licking, and even gentle biting when appropriate.

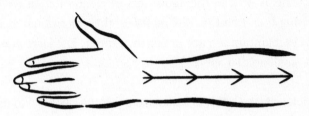

By now, the stimulating action on the energy channel in O's forearm (relating to the upper Tan Tien) will be stimulating O's pure sexual intelligence and drawing it down to mingle with the desire in O's loins (lower Tan Tien), which should move you both naturally on to a new phase of the dance.

Small golden apple

Using a fingertip, stroke the center of O's armpit, lightly and slowly, tracing circles of one-inch diameter counterclockwise on the right armpit, clockwise on the left. Trace eighteen circles in each armpit.

Ostensibly, armpits do not figure very highly in modern culture. They are thought of merely as places to be deodorized, shaved, and kept to oneself. (This handbook might change all that, however.)

The unconscious/instinctive reason why armpits are usually maintained in privacy is that in the center of each one is the beginning of the heart energy channel. The heart energy regulates the activity and tone of your mind/consciousness. This is why babies tend to keep their arms close to their body; they instinctively know not to let people fuck with their minds too early on in life.

Stimulating the armpit, as above, gains you access to the channel and positively affects the tone of O's mind. It ups the pleasure factor. This is why, in the Taoist arts of meditation, as well as tai chi, Hsing I, and Pa Kua boxing styles, the practitioner is advised to always maintain a space under the armpit, just large enough to hold a small golden apple.

To intensify the effect of stimulation, you may also like to use your tongue to trace the circles, making allowances for stubble, matted hair, chemical deodorant, and/or untoward odors that arise from toxins in the body.

Ideally, the natural scent of O's armpit will be highly sensually/sexually nourishing.

Calves

With O lying face up, slide your hands under O's calves (from the outside) and gently push your fingertips up into the fleshiest part of each calf, which is roughly in the middle of the calf, where the lower leg is widest.

Push the flesh around in circles of one-half-inch diameter, counterclockwise on the right, clockwise on the left, eighteen times.

This point on the bladder energy channel wakes up the animal spirits. Gentle stimulation increases lust levels, while strong stimulation stirs up anger from buried resentment. Only stimulate strongly if you wish to provoke an emotional (angry) catharsis. Though this is only useful if you like to fight when you fuck.

Behind the knees

Another body part you don't hear much about these days. Yet although it's hardly ever on TV or in the newspapers, the back of the knee has magical properties.

Lightly run your fingertips along the crease, from outside to inside, eighteen times on both legs. If O likes it, and you do too, use your tongue to lick slowly along the same pathway.

Stimulating the energy points along the crease sends heat into the loins.

Set things up to experience O doing this to you too, for as well as the (approximately) 110 seconds of pleasure it might give you, you may also feel how it stimulates the flow of energy in your loins as it moves from your hips into your genitals.

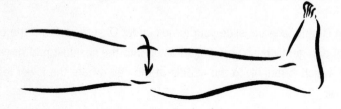

Knuckles

Stroke O's knuckles, from the joints where the fingers begin, up to the first finger joints, along the bit where little hairs grow. Do this very lightly, so as to tease the ends of the little hairs, eighteen times. You can do it on just one finger (any finger of your choice, including the thumb), on each of the fingers in turn, or on all fingers at once. You can also do it with your tongue.

This sends a mild rush of warm energy to the back of O's head and into the upper Tan Tien in center brain, which makes O's entire body relax, and in turn enables the warm energy to drop into the lower Tan Tien in the belly and fire up the loins.

Between the fingers

When holding hands with O, let your fingers play in the V-shaped spaces/webs between O's fingers (thumbs included).

When conditions permit, lick between the fingers. This sends a small pleasure shudder into O's brain.

Elbow creases

Stroke lightly and slowly along O's elbow crease, from outer edge to inner, eighteen times with your fingertips, then eighteen times with your tongue.

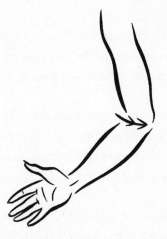

This sends a wave of energy directly into the clitoris or glans (helmet) of the penis, and is like unlocking a secret door to the genitals.

Knowing this, your passion might also lead you to kiss and suck O right in the middle of the elbow crease for a short while.

Base of the spine

Press your fingertips lightly but firmly at the base of O's spine for around seventy seconds to centralize O's consciousness in the loins. This has a stabilizing effect on O's entire energy field and helps to remind him/her where he/she is in the world, i.e., having sex with you, just in case all the stroking and licking in creases and hidden places has encouraged his/her mind to waft into never-never/always-always land.

To fully appreciate the effect, have O do this to you.

Sucking/licking between toes

Not many O's will be instantly inclined to feel comfortable with your doing this, on account of the fear that their feet might stink (especially between the little toe and next, where toxins are released).

On account of the same fear, you might like to test the smell levels by running your finger between O's little toe and the next one along, sniffing it discreetly or blatantly in accordance with the dictates of the protocol of that particular situation.

If the smell pleases you, proceed to lick between O's toes, sucking individual, pairs, and even groups of O's toes at will. Start with the little toes and work inward toward the big toes, as this encourages energy to move from the body's extremities to the sexual core. Do nine licks between each toe and suck each toe for about as long as it takes to open an oyster and swallow it.

This sends an immediate rush of warm energy up the body, through the genitals, on up through the chest/breasts and into the brain, and is quite saucy on account of its unusually intimate nature.

Be sure, however, to check first for athlete's foot so as to prevent athlete's mouth.

Using your toes

Providing you ensure adequate levels of toe/inter-toe hygiene and total freedom from fungus, it is recommended that you use your own toes to stroke the body parts belonging to O, which happen to be within easy reach of your feet, thus enabling you to perform two distinct acts of O stimulation simultaneously. [See *Toe in the Hole,* p. 154.]

Inside ankles

While French-kissing together, trace circles with your toes behind O's inner ankle bones in the natural depression formed between the ankle bone and the heel.

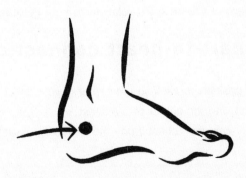

Trace eighteen circles of about one-inch diameter in a counter-clockwise direction on the left ankle, and eighteen clockwise on the right.

This sends a rush of warm energy up the back of the legs into the anal/genital region to act as a counterbalance to all the kissing action going on in the head region.

Toe in the Hole

While O is going down on you (performing fellatio/cunnilingus) and is positioned so that you are lying back, looking down at the crown of O's head as O licks/sucks, oil your big toe and work it (extremely) gently and slowly into O's asshole. Leave it there as part of the action for a while, say the time it takes to eat half a mango, then pull your toe out as (extremely) gently and slowly as you put it in. (And if O doesn't like it, you can tell O to stick it up his/her ass.)

Or simply run your toe up and down the crease between O's buttocks eighteen times (instead/as well).

In addition to being a bit rude and therefore providing a moment of potentially erotic surprise, performing this "technique" gives you a certain amount of leverage, i.e., the ability to regulate the movement of O's head (in relation to your genitals).

Heart-to-heart connection

Lying down, position yourself so the center of your chest is in full and direct contact with the center of O's chest.

Mentally relax your chest from the inside by visualizing sliding doors opening (out to the sides), so that there's nothing blocking the heart-to-heart connection.

Remain like this for as long as it takes to become restless, sometimes lying still, sometimes moving at will, but always with your focus on the connection between O's center chest (middle Tan Tien) and yours.

Pubic pinch

Pinch O lightly, i.e., delightfully, not spitefully, at the top of O's pubic bone, in the center. Pinch only with four ounces. Hold the pinch for the length of time it takes to wink at a stranger, i.e., half a second.

This point stimulates sexual fire.

On a subtle level, pubic pinching is like holding a red rag to a bull's eye, taking a crop to a trotting/cantering horse, or changing down to third at eighty. Naturally, the intensity of response is directly related to the pressure of the pinch and the length of time the pinch is sustained, as well as the intention of the pincher.

Zygomatic kisses

The zygomatic arch forms a vital part of that section of the skeletal structure that supports your face, without which your cheeks would be in grave danger of sliding off.

You may think that kissing cheeks is just for kids, cocktail parties, and aunties, however, it would be wise to open your mind on this one.

Kissing O's cheek with love and tenderness is one of the most direct ways of transmitting love directly into O's brain (upper Tan

Tien), whence it can flow downward (in the trickle-down effect) to O's heart, and radiate to fill O's entire body/being.

Kiss O's cheeks for the beauty you see there, for the subtle scent of O's life story. And don't stop yourself there. Kiss the lines at the sides of O's eyes. Lines (wrinkles) tell the story of O's life. Kiss each of O's lines as a celebration of that story.

You may even like to let loose and follow your kisses wherever they want to go, until you find yourself kissing O all over.

In any case, do up to eight kisses on each cheek, slowly, so as not to come across like a woodpecker at work, and up to four kisses on each facial line, adjusting the number of repetitions according to both the number of facial lines present and the amount of time you have to spend doing this kind of kissing. (Kidding—about the counting of facial lines, not the content.)

This endearing, affectionate action provides an effective counterbalance to rude stuff, and can produce interesting configurations of Yin and Yang in the energy flow between you when performing it at the same time as, say, sticking your finger in O's ass.

Do not be afraid to kiss O's cheek with full love because you think it might make you appear too soft, childlike, or parental. This might be the one action which transforms your sex from cold to warm.

Sucking nipple

Occasionally, you find yourself in a perfect moment. Looking out to sea from your balcony, sun on your face, not too hot, a pair of seagulls cavorting against the endless expanse of blue sky, sunlight tickling the inside of your brain, fishermen mending nets on the beach below, hands working to the rhythm of the waves. In this moment you feel no pressure, no demands. Aware that you're blending with the perfection and totality beyond time or temporal concerns, you allow yourself to feel gratitude for this perfect moment.

Beneath your balcony is an unfinished wall, a small pile of wet cement and some bricks. Three determined young men, each skilled in the ancient art of masonry, begin to bang and hammer remorselessly. Perfect moment over.

Your life is a series of moments. Moments of all shapes, sizes, hues, and tones. When you fantasize about your perfect "relationship," what you're fantasizing about is a perfect moment and/or series of moments. In real-time existence, it is these perfect moments, when they arise of themselves from the Tao, that give you the fuel, impetus, and motivation to keep going through all the other not-so-perfect moments.

As perfect moments go, there is nothing quite like finding yourself teasing, sucking, kissing, licking, and sometimes even mildly nipping the nipple and surrounding countryside of an O you love.

The ancient art of nipple stimulation revolves around encouraging O to talk to you. Not about current affairs, fashion, culture, or even spirituality. To talk to you from the heart and soul of O, in language beyond words, about love. Love and the perfect moment.

Some nipples are precocious. Some nipples are shy. Some nipples talk and even sing to you as soon as you look at them. Some nipples need coaxing over time.

This does not just vary from O to O. Often O's left nipple will have a completely different personality from O's right one. You must be observant and take the time to get to know each one. To develop a rapport. You'll probably have a favorite, as will O, and it's grand when you and O both prefer the same nipple. But don't let this encourage you to be unfair. Be sure to spend ample time dialoguing with both left and right.

Though sucking nipple is performed predominantly by boy-Os, and/or bisexual and lesbian women on O-girls, there is nothing in the rule book to prevent O-girls doing it to boy-Os with equally beneficial results. Hence the word breast in the following instructions applies to that part of O's anatomy (female or male) responsible for supporting O's nipple(s).

Take O's breast in your hand(s). In choosing which breast to take first, simply allow yourself to be pulled to one side or the other by instinct or proximity to your face. Do this with gentle authority. Take command of the breast as you would an orange (half) you were about to savor on a sunny day, or even a watermelon or mango.

Take a moment to observe the nipple in its prestimulated state. Lick slowly and lightly around the areola, as if licking around the circumference of an ice-cream cone. Observe the goose-bumping effect on the surrounding skin. Trace up to eighteen circles or more with your tongue (counterclockwise on the right nipple, clockwise on the left).

Now lick around and around the nipple itself, tracing another eighteen circles with your tongue (same direction as above). Observe any visible physiological changes in the shape, skin texture, and hue of the nipple.

Now position your open lips around the nipple, lightly and gently, with an in-and-out rolling motion of the lips, suck (like a baby sucking nectar), using the tip of your tongue to lick the nipple top each time you roll your lips under to suck the nipple in. Perform up to thirty-six lip-rolling (suck-and-release) motions, or more, then repeat the entire procedure on the other breast.

Stimulating O's nipples thus causes O noticeable heart-opening sensations and encourages great feelings of tenderness and love to flow.

Moreover, the nipples are connected energically directly to the clitoris/glans. Conducting parlance with them in this way is like winning the support of the boss's personal assistant before going in to make the big pitch.

For warming the current of sexual love, it is imperative that you suck nipple. While doing so, feel free to use your hands, feet, and other moving parts inventively to simultaneously bring pleasure to O's other breast/nipple, clitoris/glans, and/or any other part of O you fancy touching.

Worshiping ass

O's ass is a profound phenomenon. It is this very ass that supports O throughout O's life, that provides the basis upon which O's entire being sits. Moreover, it joins O's legs to O's torso (at the back, at least) and thus enables O to stand, walk, run, dance, cycle, drive a car, in short, to conduct himself/herself through daily life. O's ass is also privy to the most secret and intimate of O's doings. O's relationship with it, through lavatorial, ablutional (washing), as well as sexual activity, is sacrosanct.

For O to allow you in to this relationship, as the third part of the triangle, is an honor and should be appreciated as such.

So don't just limit your displays of appreciation for it to roughly grabbing it blind from the other side as you lay face to face with O in your arms.

Position yourself (with O's tacit consent) so you can conduct dialogue with it (face-to-face, cheek to cheek, even), just as you would with O's nipple.

As you know, an ass is usually comprised of two more or less round cheeks (buttocks) of more or less fleshy consistency, linking the back of O's legs to O's lower back, which not only house, protect, frame, and support O's anus, but can also look great in a pair of tight jeans/silk underwear/sitting on your face.

O's anus is the hidden rear entrance to the secret passageway that leads you to the mystery of O's inner world. But it's also where O's shit comes from, so it's very important to ensure that adequate ablution has occurred before attempting any serious dialogue with it. This is especially true if you intend to get fully oral in your conversation, to minimize risk of contracting hepatitis, parasites, and/or amoebas. [See *Warning and disclaimer*, p. 3.]

That notwithstanding, with both hands held together in mock-prayer position, draw your fingertips up through the crack between O's butt with four ounces, from the perineum to the sacrum (large triangular bone at the base of the spine). Separate your hands, and using your palms, stroke outward over the top of each cheek, down over the sides, in under each buttock, and back (together again) in mock-prayer position with fingertips touching O's perineum.

This comprises one cycle of the movement.

As your hands separate over the top of O's buttocks, you will notice this simultaneously causes O's buttocks to part to reveal O's asshole.

Do not be crass about this. Do not force the movement. You are not trying to force O's "O" out of hiding, merely trying to gently woo it into the light of day.

Gradually, as you repeat the movement cycle (up to thirty-six times or more), allow your hands to spread O's cheeks progressively farther apart, till (with O's continued tacit consent), O's asshole is winking at you like a flashing traffic signal.

Once you feel you have established a rapport, if you feel so compelled, draw your face closer and lick gently and slowly around the rim eighteen times counterclockwise and eighteen clockwise.

If on doing so, the (hopefully) subtle smell, taste, and general ambience is so to your liking that you wish to go deeper in dialogue, allow the tip of your tongue to lick inside the rim in circles (eighteen in each direction—if you're actually still counting).

It is best to complete, i.e., satiate both yourself and O, with all stimulation involving tongue-clitoris-vagina combinations before moving on to this, to avoid bacterial spread.

You might instead prefer (with O's ongoing tacit consent) to anally insert your finger, preoiled or naturally lubricated with O's vaginal juice, gently moving it in and out up to nine times or more, and then circling as before.

The question of whether you French kiss after you've had your tongue in O's ass is a personal one, the answer to which is usually dictated by the hygiene fixation levels, French-kissing compulsion levels, and how-rude-you-want-to-get levels of both you and O at that particular time.

However, it would be a mistake to lick O's asshole and then go straight for the French kiss just to impress O with how sexually emancipated/sophisticated you are/have become.

Licking ass is an acquired taste and is by no means obligatory, however modern you are. Some lovers have never and will never even contemplate trying it, and that's entirely up to them. Many Os, however, having experienced the sublime bliss of receiving this special attention, would think it mean of you to withhold. But if you want to be mean, be mean, if you know what I mean.

The French kiss

The French, presumably the ancient French judging by the rather primal, precultural, universal feel of this "technique," are a damn clever race when it comes to acting out matters of the heart.

There is a Wayward Taoist theory/myth that the art of the French kiss was brought here originally by aliens, who on meeting the French, and being suitably impressed by the elegant way they kissed one another on both cheeks, as well as their apparent adroitness at handling the various conundrums that arise with affairs of the heart, decided to pass on this valuable method of exchanging sexual love (and saliva). Eventually, with the universal spread of all things French—haute couture, fine perfume, joi de vivre, etc.—the French kiss finally gave in and went global.

In other words, you don't need to be French to do this properly, just as you don't need to be Chinese or even Taoist. You just need a pair of lips, a tongue, and an O similarly equipped who wants to French-kiss you.

French-kissing, involving the interpenetration of tongues into mouths, means far more, however, than simply sticking your tongue down O's throat.

Place your face in proximity to O's, so that your lips meet. Let your lips meet gently at first. Start with your lips slightly parted.

Take time to feel the joy of closeness. Move your lips in a gentle kissing motion until you feel O's mouth open a little more (of itself—no forcing).

Relax and soften your tongue. Breathing in and out softly through your nose, slowly lead your tongue to penetrate into O's mouth, avoiding but not being scared of O's teeth, until your (two) tongues meet.

Gently lead your tongue back out again and regroup. When you feel ready, repeat penetration until your tongues meet again, this time spending a little longer together. You may want to pull out once more so you can penetrate again, or you may find yourself swept on strong currents of desire to let go, relax, and suck your tits off in a wild fandango of dancing tongues, teasing, pressing, urging, darting forth, retreating, circling, searching, and finding. Finding that you love this O so much you want to stay with her/him forever (and drive each other mad). Or you may just want to keep French-kissing for a while longer.

In which case, you might notice the inherent Yin-Yangness of the situation. Your tongue advances, O's tongue retreats. Advancing is Yang, retreating is Yin. For the balance between these to be maintained, ensure that the action isn't all going one way. Dance a little in O's mouth, retreat and let O dance awhile in yours. Don't seek to overpower or suffocate with your tongue. Be delicate about it. Enjoy kissing around O's mouth too. The small crack at the side of the mouth, the indentation (philtrum) running down from the nose to the upper lip, the side of the lip, side of the tongue, under the tongue, kiss, suck, let your tongues dance in a frenzy of celebration for desire fulfilled.

Sharing your saliva is like sharing the juice of your soul, for that moment (so remember your oral hygiene). There is nothing lightweight about the French kiss, which is why it often gets you into so much trouble.

French-kissing, sometimes referred to as getting off with someone, is traditionally associated with the start of the love story, the reenactment of which plays a crucial part in sustaining that love over the long term. A love story without the passion both engendered by and which engenders the full French kiss (at least from time to time) has died. (You *know* that.)

When you and O are in a full face-to-face genitally penetrative embrace, be sure to spend ample time doing the French kiss as this facilitates direct transmission of chi from upper Tan Tien to upper Tan Tien and is also essential to conduct the chi between you during the enactment of Whooshing the Chi.

[See *Whooshing the Chi*, p. 199, and *Connecting your Three (Six) Tan Tiens*, p. 197.]

Hand jobs

This is (primarily) for O-girls dealing with boy-Os.

Every man likes to jerk off in his own particular/peculiar way. Your role is not necessarily to replicate that. It is to jerk him off in your own unique way custom-adapted (over time) to please that particular O. In other words, you must jerk him off in a way he'll never forget and which he can't do for himself (or he might as well do it himself).

There is no universally correct way to jerk a man off. There are, however, with the exception of dealing with an out-and-out brute, one or two universal things *not* to do.

You should not grab hold of his dick as if clutching the gearshift of an off-road sports utility vehicle falling off a cliff, to slam it into reverse.

Nor should you attempt to grab it after prolonged trapeze, rope-climbing practice, or any other manual activity that has caused excessive callusing of the palms.

The penis must be taken gently but firmly in your hand. Not fearfully, in loving awe perhaps, but not timidly or gingerly. Apply only four ounces of pressure. Don't get stuck on holding it. Stroke it delicately up and down the length of its noble shaft, along the back, front, and sides. Use the tips of your fingers like feathers. Don't be functional about it. Transmit love through your hands and fingertips.

Don't isolate the penis. Let your fingertips stroke (very lightly) over his balls, under them, and into his perineum.

What you're looking for is to establish a relationship with O's dick. You've got to get it/him to talk to you. You've got to become allies. After all, he's O's closest friend. Like any wild animal with a mind of its own, you have to break him in gently. Gain his trust. Hence the need to go in confidently. But you must be extremely sensitive.

Penises, like vaginas, can get sore easily from excess friction. So always make initial contact softly to gauge O's idea of four ounces. If you have some oil/lubrication to hand it might be helpful to avail yourself of it at this point. Otherwise/anyway feel free to use your own vaginal fluid and/or saliva by first collecting it in your hand(s).

(The following is for when O's dick is erect, but can be easily adapted when wishing to perform manual alchemy on a flaccid one.)

Arrange yourself so that you're perfectly comfortable. Relax your shoulders, elbows, and wrists. Breathe. Take hold of O's dick as though taking hold of a ceremonial mace and smooth the lubrication you have chosen to use into the shaft, being sure to cover the entire surface area evenly. Apply enough pressure for your hand to move the outer skin against the shaft, but not so much that you actually pull the skin, which is very similar to the delicate skin around your eyes.

There are four sides to a penis: left, right, front, and back. I need to clarify front and back here. When the penis is flaccid, the front, i.e., the part you see when looking at O's full-frontal aspect, becomes the back when O's penis becomes erect. And the back, i.e., the part you don't see (the underside) becomes the front. To avoid confusion, I'm calling the underside-when-flaccid aspect, the underside (funnily enough), and the other side, the topside. Left and right remain the same.

Run your fingers up the midline of the underside from base to tip, and down the topside from tip to base eighteen times, going very lightly, especially over the top of the head (helmet), as if running your fingers over gold leaf.

On an energetic/reflexive level this stimulates energy to Scoop the Loop up and down the spinal column to which these energy lines correspond, thus helping rebalance Yin and Yang (bet you never thought giving someone a hand job could be quite so medicinal).

Now, either using both hands or thumb and forefinger of one, stroke likewise up both left and right sides simultaneously from base to tip eighteen times. This builds up an expectant sexual charge and will make O wish (possibly fervently) for you to put some more lubrication on your hand and take hold of his dick with conviction. An act which you should not hesitate to perform, starting off by holding the middle third of the shaft and moving the flesh against it in a steady up and down rhythm.

Check that the shoulder, elbow, and wrist of your active hand are relaxed, your body is comfortably positioned, and your breath is regulated and flowing freely.

Do not start at a fast pace. Begin slowly and attempt only to hold

the tempo steady, moving up and down the shaft about an inch upward and downward of the halfway point.

As your strokes grow more confident, allow your hand to move up
and down over more distance until your movement covers the entire
length.

There is a given moment at which the tempo starts taking you
faster of itself. Wait until you feel this before accelerating. At which
point you might like to decide between you if this is intended to
make O ejaculate or not. If so, be sure to maintain constant pressure with your hand and to keep your arm relaxed to facilitate double-
time piston motion, if required, for as long as necessary. Be extremely
tempo-sensitive when O ejaculates, as different boy-Os need you to
decelerate/stop the stimulation at different times; some as soon as
they squirt, others not until they've squeezed out every last drop, and
others somewhere in-between.

However, when employing your hand thus as merely part of the
greater sexual dance, which is more often than not the case, you
will need to cease all manual stimulation before O's penis, and especially glans (helmet), starts to go a bit purplish and swell that
extra bit (as it does).

It can be both usefully informative and socially entertaining to
employ the verbal communication mode in order to ascertain the
exact details of O's requirements, likes and dislikes, apropos being
tossed off. And, of course, vice versa.

And just as verbal communication is a two-way thing, so is mutual touching. To which end you will occasionally find yourself
performing this technique, while O simultaneously performs its female equivalent on you.

O-girl, manual clitoral stimulation thereof

This is mostly for boy-Os when dealing with a clitoris.

Except in sexual emergencies, never rush straight to the clitoris. Every attempt must be made to approach it indirectly, through the agency of the aforementioned "techniques." Permission must first be granted and graciously received before wandering into the holy of holies, the inner temple. You don't just go wading in, tweak it once or twice (if you can find it in the first place), and expect that to open any doors, other than with the most brutish of O-girls.

Approach O's clitoris with respect. Not with reverence, after all it's only a clitoris, but with respect. Respect, from the Latin, *re*: again and *spectare*: to look at, means literally to look at something again/afresh, as in truly notice it. To do this, actually have a look at O's clitoris, I mean with your eyes. Not like a doctor (not a medical one anyway), but like a proper lover should. With desire, curiosity, fascination, and relish.

If you can't see where it is, ask O to show you with her finger. Feel it with your finger. Like penises, clitorises come in all manner of shapes and sizes, but all generally nestle beneath a little hood right at the front way in/out of the vagina, at the back of the pubic bone. Like a small semihard cactus button it sits at the core of O's core and is intimately involved, on a vibrational level at least, in everything she does and experiences. You could say it's her soul-button, because the pleasure it gives her is the deepest pleasure of the soul.

To which end, if you wish, or find it incumbent on yourself, to partake of this particular mode of pleasure-giving, it is well to first lubricate your finger by gently inserting it between O's labia (vaginal lips) and scooping out some juice to use as lubrication. You might find it instructive to first watch O do this to herself, as this is how O-girls generally masturbate.

Relax your shoulder, elbow, and wrist. Check you've placed your body in the optimum position for comfort and ease of movement. Breathe freely and deeply. Place your lubricated (optional) fingertip on O's clitoris, using only four ounces. Do this slowly, gently, sensitively, yet firmly and with conviction. Don't try to give the impression of being an old hand. Be vulnerable, humble, yet proud in the face of the Unfathomable Female Mystery (UFM).

Move the fleshy hood from side to side against the clitoris with your fingertip, in a side-to-side slow-tempo vibrating style, moving but a millimeter each way, while you count up to five breath cycles (in and out), constantly checking for visual, audio, or kinetic indications of whether or not she likes what you're doing.

Now move the flesh back and forth in similar vibrating style for a similar number of breaths.

By general consent or plain intuition, you may find yourself speeding up so that your hand is vibrating like an electric drill (or handheld vibrator). When this occurs pay special attention to relaxing your shoulder, elbow, and wrist and breathing slowly, deeply, and freely to prevent your hand cramping and thus losing speed and intensity at a crucial moment.

With your forefinger, circle slowly around the top of O's clitoris eighteen times counterclockwise and eighteen times clockwise.

You can combine this to great orgasmic effect with other "techniques"/moves such as sticking the finger(s) of your free hand in

O's vagina and/or anus, the French kiss, sucking nipple, penile penetration (vaginal or anal), and even Toe in the Hole, if you're agile enough, or simply have O do it to herself while you do everything else.

However, never approach the clitoris with a goal in mind. Remember this is the feminine, the Yin, the formless, lateral state without goals. Otherwise you're in danger of finding yourself with a severely cramped arm vibrating at high speed, praying, "Oh, please make her come now!" while you rub her numb.

Meeting belly

Just because O's belly hasn't got many secret bits on it, other than the semisecret belly button, doesn't mean it's boring.

O's belly houses O's lower Tan Tien, that field of divine energy that regulates and fuels O's desire. O-girl's belly also houses her sacred womb, i.e., potential people-carrier. You came from a womb. Womb is a universal concept, and here you have one (boy-O), a living representative of the universal archetype, all covered in soft/firm, round/flat belly, right before your very eyes.

Bury your face in O's belly. Just be there for a while. Let your cheek rest against it. Love it as you would the center of life itself.

Look at O's navel. That was once the terminus of the umbilical cord that gave O life. Honor that.

Kiss O's belly button again and again (no more than eighty-one times).

This act of love and appreciation for O's existence also acts as an effective prelude to oral sex maneuvers, will usually cause penises to become engorged, i.e., go stiff, and furthermore gives you an indication, when dallying with a newfound O, of whether you'd find the natural scent of their "special place" too hot to handle at closer quarters.

Blow jobs

Now there's a topic.

This is mostly for O-girls when confronted by a penis (erect or flaccid), which it behooves them to excite by means other than manual or vaginal, i.e., orally.

According to Wayward Taoist mythology, blow jobs earned their moniker from being just that. Blow jobs. Blowing air over the erect penis was only superseded by licking and sucking in later times as people lost the natural way and grew more greedy.

Unfortunately for those who made their living from "playing the jade flute," once people had tasted the pleasures of fully bringing mouth to organ, they found it difficult to return to their former saliva-free ways.

Nevertheless, it is considered important by Waywards the world over for the sexual-spiritual development of O-girls that they practice and hopefully gain a degree of proficiency in the ancient art of "playing the jade flute."

Position yourself comfortably between O's legs in such a way that you are looking at his penis at close quarters.

Taking hold of it gently in one hand, cup his testicles softly in the other.

Take in a comfortably long lungful of air, and be sure to keep topping it up as you would when playing a conventional flute.

Blow along the midline of the underside from base to tip eighteen times.

Now blow along the midline of the topside from tip to base eighteen times.

No advantage will be gained by speed. Do not rush this, but play it as a slow, authoritative solo (*piano-piano*).

Now blow up and down the length of the left side of the shaft and then the right.

Now blow over the balls, gently lifting them with your hand as you do, so you can blow beneath them and into the perineum.

Now repeat the entire sequence once or twice or until you get dizzy/bored.

When this is performed correctly with aplomb, grace, and finesse, the sensations of pleasure engendered, not only in and around the penis but throughout the entire organism, are truly sublime. This is one of the few ways to make a man come in midair. (Immaculate ejaculation.)

Providing you stop short of that, however, you are now free to bring your lips, tongue, and oral cavity to bear on the situation.

Position yourself so that your mouth is side-on to the shaft of O's penis. Arrange your upper body so that the back of your neck is relaxed and elongated, i.e., not contracted or tense. Breathe slowly and softly through your nose. Relax your jaw. Relax the root of your tongue and soften the tip with your mind.

Take hold of the base of the shaft with one hand and cup the scrotum with the other.

Using four ounces, lick slowly and purposefully along the midline of the underside from base to tip, and down the topside from tip to base, employing a hardly discernible side-to-side wiggling motion of the tongue, up to eighteen times or more.

Now reposition yourself so that you're face-to-face with the underside of the shaft, and, moving your tongue from side to side for enough in each direction to span the entire width of the shaft, gradually work your way up from the base to the tip and back down again, up to eighteen times or more, or until your neck stiffens or you get bored.

Now, gently lifting O's balls, use your tongue tip to trace small circles on one ball at a time, counterclockwise on the right one and clockwise on the left, nine times on each side.

Placing your tongue tip under O's scrotum, circle it nine times counterclockwise and nine times clockwise on O's perineum (Gate of Mortality).

Now lick from the perineum, up through the narrow gap between O's testicles and along the underside of the shaft to the tip, using the same small side-to-side tongue wiggling motion as before. Repeat this upwardly directed lick up to eighteen times or more, or until you can feel O gagging for you to take his penis in your mouth.

Relax your jaw fully. Breathe softly but deeply through your nose. Place your lips carefully over the glans (helmet) of O's penis. Open your jaw as wide as you can to prevent your teeth inadvertently nipping or in any way causing abrasion to the shaft. Slowly, as if sucking a delicious Popsicle on a sweltering summer's day, begin to suck the glans.

Roll your lips inward and use your tongue to draw the glans into your mouth. Roll your lips outward to release it, thus instigating a Yin-Yang, in-out motion of penis and mouth. Repeat this on the glans up to thirty-six times, remaining vigilant about your teeth at all times.

Relax the back of your mouth and throat. Check that your neck is not stiffening. Breathe deeply and softly through your nose. Continue sucking O's cock as you were, gradually taking it in farther and farther until it's as if O is actually having intercourse with your mouth.

For this motion to blossom fully, you must surrender yourself to what's going on, i.e., offer up your head to O's pleasure. Hence the phrase, giving head.

At this point it may be wise to ascertain (somehow) whether the intention is to make O come or to stop and let things develop along other less one-sided lines. And if it's the former, to decide whether you wish O to finish in your mouth—and whether you're going to swallow—and to proceed accordingly. If you wish O to come but *don't* wish to swallow his sperm, have a tissue handy in which to discreetly and daintily spit out the sperm as inoffensively as you can, or have your hand ready to jerk him off at the same tempo as the sucking, as soon as you take your mouth away.

If, however, you wish to move the dance on, let O complete up to thirty-six thrusts in and out and then slowly move your mouth away.

To complete the circle, French-kiss as a gesture of share and share alike.

Cunnilingus, the joys of

This is mostly for boy-O's, who, when staring a vagina straight in the eye feel an inclination to put lip to lip and eat some pussy, as it were.

Cunnilingus comes from the Latin *cunnus* and *lingere* and means, literally, cunt and tongue. However, it also involves the use of lips and sometimes even the chin.

Having ascertained that the taste and scent of O's vagina is to your liking, by either kissing her belly or putting a finger inside and sniffing it (discreetly or otherwise), position yourself between O's legs.

Relax the back of your neck and upper body. Relax your jaw and soften your tongue. Breathe slowly and deeply through your nose, immersing yourself in the atmosphere.

Using the fingertips of both hands, gently part O's labia. Let the tip of your tongue dart deftly between them, scoop out some fluid, and draw it upward onto O's clitoris. Now circle your tongue tip slowly, around the clitoris eighteen times counterclockwise and eighteen times clockwise to stir the sexual fire.

Now put your tongue tip back between the lips and scoop out some more fluid, which mixed with your saliva, produces a fine lubricant, and run your tongue tip back and forth on the top of O's clitoris thirty-six times at a medium tempo.

Scoop some more fluid, this time allowing your tongue to penetrate more deeply into O's vagina, and wiggle your tongue tip from side to side on the top of O's clitoris thirty-six times at medium tempo.

Scoop some more fluid, this time penetrating as far as your tongue will go, and placing your lips over O's clitoris, sucking it gently while allowing O to simultaneously rub herself against your chin if she should so desire. Suck for the time it takes to complete nine full breath cycles.

Now let your tongue slide back between O's labia and penetrate as deeply as it will go. Use your tongue like a penis, darting in and out, as though sucking a sherbet fountain. Lick around the walls of O's vagina, exploring everywhere.

If you (both) want, you can return to the start of the entire cunnilingual sequence and begin again now.

If O should come during this sequence, be highly sensitive and alert to her slightest signal as to whether she wants you to accelerate, decelerate, stop, or simply carry on as you were. It could be helpful to agree on prearranged verbal signals such as speed up, slow down, stop, or keep going. Otherwise, feel free to ask her between mouthfuls.

Having completed part or all of the above cunnilingual sequence, your passion may lead you to immerse yourself fully in the gobblesome act of eating O's pussy. This requires that you use your entire mouth and all auxiliary oral equipment other than teeth to literally devour O's privates, as if feasting on the universal Yin. It is impossible and unnecessary to adequately describe correct eating "technique." Some boy-Os eat their food like pigs, or worse. Others eat their food like noblemen. Obviously, the more refined your table manners, the more refined a response you'll get from O.

Do not overstimulate O's genitals to the point of numbness or pain (hers or yours). You may find the root of your tongue feels sore or overworked later on. To avoid tongue strain and to strengthen your tongue to increase inherent pleasure-giving factor levels, practice the following on your own every morning, noon, and night.

Sitting comfortably, breathing deeply and slowly through your nose, circle your tongue around the back of your gums, behind your teeth, eighteen times counterclockwise and eighteen times clockwise. Now circle it around the outside of your gums eighteen times in each direction. Finally, knock your upper and lower teeth together (gently) thirty-six times.

Not only will this improve your cunnilingual skills, it will improve your French-kissing technique, help heal and/or prevent gum disease, help clarify your enunciation, and tone your endocrine system and specifically your pituitary gland.

Once you've become comfortable with all the above and wish to gain a different perspective on the matter, try it out lying on your back, head supported by a firm, friendly pillow/cushion/ I Ching, and have O sit on your face.

Soixante-neuf

The French have been responsible for making many ancient oriental ideas universally famous. The most commonly used Western term to describe energy channels, for example, is the French word meridian, meaning channel. Another example is the French kiss. Even condoms are affectionately known as French-letters. But perhaps the best known is the ancient art of soixante-neuf.

Nothing describes/depicts the dance of Yin and Yang as eloquently as two Os engaged in soixante-neuf (69), more or less a dead ringer for the Yin-Yang symbol.

Performing 69 with O is the most direct way of balancing Yin and Yang between you, and is recommended before penile insertion occurs.

Boy-O sucks Yin from O-girl and O-girl sucks Yang from boy-O in one of three ways. Namely, boy-O on top, O-girl on top, or both lying on their sides. Quite often, you find yourself rolling/squirming from one to the other.

Soixante-neuf often occurs when boy-O is going down on O-girl, with O-girl on her back, head adequately supported by cushions, if required. After a while, he realigns the north–south axis of his body to position himself with genitals directly over O's oral region. Kneeling over O's face, he spreads his legs and lowers his genitals onto O's mouth, who then proceeds to lick and suck his Yang, pulling his (hopefully, at this stage) erect penis back when necessary to fit it in her mouth, while simultaneously using her hands to grab his ass.

At the same time, boy-O is licking and sucking her in similar fashion, using his hands to cup and lift her buttocks to facilitate the tongue action, as required.

The pair may then roll sideways into the intermediate position, spend some time with this new perspective and then roll into O-girl on top position.

Now boy-O is lying on his back, head amply supported by cushions, licking and sucking O in comfort and *she* gets the stiff neck.

While thus engaged, use your hands and fingers to substantiate the action. For example, insert your finger in vagina and/or anus, and/or stroke O and/or yourself off while simultaneously licking and sucking.

When performed gracefully, soixante-neuf can bring hours of delicate pleasure to you and O. You may find yourself mimicking/mirroring each other's moves in a similar way to ballroom dancing, or you may find that each gets lost in his/her own world of other-sex genital exploration/worship. But probably, as with most things in real-time life, it'll be a combination.

Putting two fingers up

This is mostly for boy-Os who wish to stimulate the flow of O's vaginal juices, increase O's level of sexual receptivity, and specifically to ease the passage of his penis prior to insertion.

This is similar in style to a reversed peace/victory sign, but different in execution, in that the two fingers are usually held together.

While most prefer clitoral masturbation, some O-girls are more sexually stimulated by having two fingers up.

Positioning yourself so as to avoid any unnecessary wrist strain, insert first one finger and then the next, slowly and gently between O's labia. Allow your fingers to penetrate half an inch or so, moving them in and out slowly against the vaginal opening nine times.

Now let them slide in as far as they'll go, just once, and pull them back to the opening.

Thrice repeat this procedure of nine shallow finger thrusts and one deep thrust.

Now circle your fingers at full insertion depth around O's vaginal walls nine times counterclockwise and nine times clockwise, with your fingertips reaching the tip of O's uterus, if possible.

Keep your finger action light, active, and sensitive, and be alert to internal physical signals from O's vagina, as well as verbal signals to ascertain whether she likes what you're doing.

If, after completing the above sequence, you both agree this is the moment for penile penetration, you can then use your fingers to open the vagina in order to ease your penis's ingress.

Scratching

It is quite common for girls (and some boys) in the throes of sexual ecstasy, to compulsively scratch O with her (or his) fingernails.

Except when specifically mutually agreed by prior arrangement, scratching should be kept relatively light to avoid drawing blood, as this level of pain-sharpness can be off-putting unless O is overtly masochistic and/or exceptionally thick-skinned.

To keep your scratching enjoyable, attend to your manicure in such a way that the ends of your nails are slightly blunted/buffed, i.e., not like razor blades.

As any good Taoist DJ will tell you, only scratch with four ounces.

Use your scratching, *like* a DJ does, to provide moments of rhythmic intensification to accentuate the beat of the penile thrust.

Most scratching occurs on shoulders, back (upper and lower), and possibly the arms, while O-girl has boy-O inside her.

Scratching, like acupuncture, is a powerful way to move chi in a hurry.

Using the fingernails of both hands, reach around and scratch softly down either side of O's spine, from the back of the head to the sacrum. Separate your hands and scratch outward over each hip/buttock to the sides, then up the sides of O's belly and chest/breast, circumventing shoulder blades and ending up with your nails once more on the back of O's head. This comprises one cycle. Repeat up to three times, slowly and delicately for best results.

Biting

Biting in its extreme form is used by humans, animals, and certain reptiles, fish, and insects to chew into something, animal flesh, for example, in order to eat it.

In its not so extreme forms, biting can be used during the sexual dance to stimulate the flow of O's sexual energy.

Biting is similar to inserting an acupuncture needle in its effect on the human organism, and acts directly on O's energy field. The energy with which you bite is the energy you transmit directly to

O. So, never bite with spite. Never bite so hard you cause bruising or disfiguration (unless specifically mutually agreed, for whatever reason, by prior arrangement). Merely nip. Gently, gently.

Nip the nipple. Nip the clitoris. Nip the scrotum. Nip the side of the penile shaft. Nip the labia. Nip the buttock. Nip the breast. Nip the shoulder, front and back. Nip the upper arm. Nip the back of the hand. Nip the calf. Nip the inner thigh. Nip the belly.

Perform only one nip in each location, remembering at all times to nip lightly. And note that having your clitoris, penile shaft, labia, scrotum, or nipple nipped is similar in intensity to having your lower eyelid nipped, so be sensitive with your teeth. [See *Warning and disclaimer*, p. 3.]

Nipping is an effective tool to prevent the dance getting too marshmallowy. Excess nipping should be avoided, however, to prevent yourself coming over like a demented mosquito (or worse).

Biting, while simultaneously sucking, produces a small bruise known as a hickey. The sensation is like cupping in Chinese medicine, quite pleasant and stimulating. However, you can only really get away with sporting a love bite in public up to the age of twenty and a half, or thereabouts, so when administering one to an O over that age, be sure to plant it somewhere other than the neck or hard-to-conceal body parts.

Pinching

Pinching plays an almost identical role to nipping/biting, but can be used more effectively as a rapid-response mechanism on account of the fact that the hand moves quicker than the head.

If, for example, you sense an urgent need to suddenly stimulate

O's energy field and do not have adequate time to move your head into place to execute a nip, simply move your hand(s) to the desired location(s), and, taking a small portion of the relevant flesh between thumb and forefinger, gently but suddenly pinch with four ounces.

This sort of maneuver is a useful way to wake O from the kind of trance that leads to boring, secondhand repetitive sexual moves and agendas, and can be helpful in breaking patterns, thus preventing long-term sexual ruts.

As with biting, never pinch so hard that you cause disfiguration or bruising (unless you both want it that way).

Pinch boy-O's perineum firmly if you think he's going to suddenly ejaculate, in order to bang shut his Gate of Mortality.

Pinch around O's groin to stir O's deep animal passions.

Pinch the top of O's wrist to make O generally more responsive and sexually alert.

Pinch the back of O's neck, just behind O's ears, below where the neck joins the skull, to break stale patterning.

Pinch O's ass (because it's irresistible sometimes).

Tickling

Tickling is a way of overexciting the nerves. Tickling when taken too far for too long is irritating, however. In extreme conditions, it *can* make you insane. Tickling an opponent to death is an actual Taoist martial art.

Keep tickling to a minimum. Use it only to lighten things up a little if O's getting too earnest about everything and needs reminding to loosen up and giggle a bit.

Therefore, unless specifically requested to do otherwise, avoid tickling in favor of good, honest stroking or scratching.

Tickling teases the nerves on account of the speed and pressure with which you pass your tickling instrument over the site you're tickling. Fast, light movement over the surface of the skin produces the tickling itch. Fast, deep movement causes pain. Slow, light movement causes pleasure. Slow, deep movement also causes pleasure.

You should choose your preference between you (and stop all that tickling shit, will ya?).

Fucking, positions thereof

There is no emphasis on acrobatic sex in either Wayward or Traditional Taoism.

Although combinations and nuances are myriad, positions for fucking an O of the opposite sex are essentially limited to the following:

O-girl on top, with legs open, lying front to front on boy-O.

O-girl on top, with legs open, sitting up while boy-O lies down.

O-girl on top, with legs open, sitting up front to front with boy-O (who's sitting up as well), with knees crossed, legs spread, legs straight, or sitting in a chair or on the side of the bed, etc.

O-girl on top, lying with legs closed on top of boy-O's legs, front to front, thigh to thigh.

O-girl on top, lying with legs closed between boy-O's open legs.

O-girl on top, sitting with legs closed and knees on boy-O's chest.

O-girl on top, sitting with legs open and back to boy-O.

O-girl on top, sitting with legs closed, back to boy-O and knees on boy-O's thighs.

Boy-O on top, lying front to front, with O-girl's legs open.

Boy-O on top, lying front to front, with O-girl's legs wrapped round his lower, middle, or upper back.

Boy-O on top, lying front to front, with O-girl's legs closed and his open.

Boy-O on top, suspended in a yogic push-up position, limiting contact to the pelvic region.

O-girl and boy-O standing (in a shop doorway), front to front, with one of O-girl's legs wrapped around boy-O's waist.

Boy-O standing strong in "horse stance," feet three feet apart, knees bent, back straight, supporting O-girl, both of whose legs are wrapped around his waist.

Boy-O standing front to back with O-girl, as in doing it from behind, with O-girl standing straight-legged, legs together or spread, but bent over (the kitchen table, for instance).

O-girl on hands and knees with boy-O kneeling behind her.

O-girl on elbows and knees with boy-O kneeling behind her.

O-girl on knees with face buried in pillow/cushion, moaning loudly, and boy-O kneeling.

O-girl lying on front with boy-O lying face-down on top of her.

O and O lying on their sides, front to front, with O-girl's upper leg wrapped around boy-O's waist.

O and O lying on their sides, front to back, legs closed, boy-O coming in from behind.

And unless I'm suffering from severe sexual amnesia or indeed am in possession of a gaping great hole in my education/experience, that's about it. That is, if you discount doing it through a hole in a sheet and other such games.

Feel free to move between postures at will, according to the Tao of the dance at the time, or remain in only one posture for the rest of your lives together.

Certain postures allow deeper penetration than others, but there is no universal rule on which is which, on account of the widely varying anatomical placement of everybody's sexual organs.

Certain postures are more sexy than others, but only for you at that time with that particular O. Postures are like chemistry, their import/value changes with the circumstances.

However, it's true to say that doing it from behind, and hearing O-girl scream with pleasure into the pillow as you pump and thrust, can get pretty bestial sometimes. While for the more spiritual purposes of Whooshing the Chi and other inner-alchemical chops, front to front with full mouth-to-mouth, chest-to-chest, and belly-to-belly connection is essential.

It is unnecessary to describe any of the positions in more depth because our concern is the principle common to all positions, of meditating while you move.

One amusing Wayward Taoist game is to "work" (nice work if you can get it) your way through all of the postures/positions and variations in any one session in any sequence you like, without boy-O's penis ever once slipping all the way out (of O-girl's vagina).

Moving gracefully between positions

Moving from one position to the next without boy-O slipping out is a bit like a game of Twister, and requires a certain amount of dexterity, care, flexibility, and strength.

Moving between positions is best done slowly, deliberately, and mindfully, so as to maintain both the physical and psycho-energic connection between you and O at all times during the dance, lest Yin and Yang become separated at the wrong moment.

When face-to-face, with one O on top and one O underneath, if you wish to change over, use the following guidelines.

Whichever O is recumbent underneath must open his/her legs, wrap them around the upper O's legs, thus locking pelvises in position, and pull upper O's chest close, so that the two bodies are pressed together with upper O's arms around lower O's upper body.

Lower O then pushes upward and to the left with the right elbow, and with one deft motion, grasping hold of upper O's back with the left arm, flips the pair of them over. It takes some practice to discover the fulcrum point at which the entire mass flips, but is only a matter of balance and intention. Once you've got it, it's as easy as falling off your log.

When boy-O is inside O-girl from behind and wishes to come around to the front in order to be face-to-face with O-girl, it goes like this.

Boy-O sits back on his heels, knees spread well apart, pulling O-girl down carefully into his lap. He then leans his upper body back, takes O-girl's upper body firmly in his hands, and literally rotates her (clockwise if he's right-handed, counterclockwise if he's left), moving her upper body slowly enough for her to lift first one leg and then the other over his head as she comes all the way around until she's sitting face-to-face with him.

When boy-O is face-to-face with O-girl and wishes to get behind her, he first assumes/moves into the recumbent position (underneath) with her sitting on top. He then reaches across, takes hold of her right lower leg with his right hand, and pulls her leg over his head to the right, thus enabling her to rotate her torso through the horizontal until she's sitting on him with her back to him.

He then sits up with her in his lap and, moving the pair of them slightly out to the side, swings them both into the forward kneeling position.

Try these out, following the instructions carefully, not only as a way of sharpening your intellect but also for the hours of fun you may (or may not) have.

All other variations follow from these basic moves and can be easily discovered on your own (with O) in your own time.

If at any time boy-O's penis slips out, smack him hard on the wrist (kidding)—don't get upset about it. It's only a game. Often it just means it's time to do some of the other weird shit in this book, or simply to stop (have a cigarette) and go to sleep.

Sacred entry

O's vagina is representative of the archetypal Vagina of the World, i.e., the feminine archetype or Big Yin. Entry therein is a sacred business and must be approached with respect by boy-Os and O-girls alike.

On entering, remain at the entrance until invited in farther. It's like waiting in the hall/lobby/foyer while the butler tells madam you're here. To rush straight into her private chambers would simply be bad manners.

In any case, you need time to stop and get your bearings. Time to appreciate the wonder of all the new sensations around you. It's like letting your spaceship dock before charging through the hatch into the mothership.

This pause allows the chi to settle before you really start stirring it up, and is especially helpful in preventing sudden surprise ejaculation.

Count at least thirty-six breath cycles, breathing in unison with O if possible, before beginning any form of pelvic motion.

This stillness can be achieved either by prior arrangement (by phone or e-mail, etc.), by on-the-spot verbal communication, as in, "Stay still for a moment, honey," or by manual communication, as in taking firm hold of O's hips with your hands and temporarily locking them into position. Of these, saying what you want at the time is usually best. Or you can write a note.

Shallow thrust

(This is easier to describe from boy-O's perspective.)

After thirty-six breath cycles or so, when you've begun to feel acclimatized to your new surroundings, push your dick in slowly to the depth of one inch only. Pause for a millisecond and pull it back to the entrance again. Pause for another millisecond and repeat, completing thirty-six shallow thrusts. On the thirty-sixth thrust, remain perfectly still, with your dick in at the depth of one inch only.

This Sexual Stillpoint allows O-girl to massage the sides of your penis with the walls of her vagina, an art she can easily acquire by practicing the Big Squeeze on a daily basis. [See *The Sexual Stillpoint*, p. 191, and *The Big Squeeze*, p. 117.]

Medium thrust

Pull back from one inch to the entrance, and, breathing slowly so as not to accelerate the tempo of your energy and thrust, slowly push in past the one-inch mark to a depth of three and a half inches. Pause for a moment and pull back out to the entrance. Pause for a moment and repeat. Complete thirty-six cycles and on the thirty-sixth, stay still at a depth of three and a half inches, resisting all temptation to go deeper just yet.

If you're doing this right and the chemistry's all in place, O-girl should be giving you vocal indications by now that she's having a damn good time, or at least good enough to bother to fake the rest.

Full thrust

Pull back to the entrance. Pause for a moment to gather yourself and regulate your breathing. Now push in slowly and deliberately all the way to the end of your dick or her vagina, whichever's nearer. Pause for a moment (while O-girl gasps either through good manners or genuine delight), and pull back out to the entrance. Pause for a moment, regulate your breath, and repeat.

Complete thirty-six cycles (if you can, without coming) and on the thirty-sixth, remain perfectly still, all the way in, allowing the walls of O's vagina to massage your penis. If you find this internal stimulation too strong at the moment, ask her to stop for a second or two.

Mixing up your thrusts

Once you're familiar with the basic thrust patterns, try mixing them up in the following manner.

Pull back to the entrance. Do five shallow thrusts followed by one medium thrust. Repeat this cycle eighteen times.

Pull back to one inch. Breathe, collect yourself, and do five medium thrusts followed by one shallow. Repeat this cycle nine times.

Now do five medium thrusts followed by one full thrust. Repeat this nine times.

Now pull back to the entrance and do nine shallow thrusts followed by one full (solid, bang her on the head from the inside) thrust.

Repeat this cycle eighteen times (if you can without coming) and stop still fully inside.

If at any time you think you're going to succumb to sudden surprise ejaculation (SSE), immediately pull back to the entrance, remain perfectly still, requesting O-girl to do likewise, and perform the Big Squeeze once, twice, or even thrice.

Alternatively, you could try riding the shudders. [See below.]

Naturally it would take a deep level of diligence and commitment to the cause to be able to follow these instructions precisely or anywhere near precisely, but if from time to time you try out the general idea, you won't be sorry.

Riding the shudders

There is a point during the climb up the slope of no return, when boy-O's perineum starts to pulse strongly with the involuntary squeeze-and-release pumping action necessary to make him ejaculate. If, at this point, he wishes to prevent ejaculation and doesn't feel in the mood for a Big Squeeze, he can try riding the shudders instead.

At the point at which you first feel the involuntary pumping action begin, simply go with the rhythm of the pulsing, exaggerating it by consciously contracting and releasing, i.e., pulling up and letting down the perineum in time with every involuntary contraction and release motion, thereby mastering it by conscious control.

You thus take command of the flow of sexual energy and are able more easily to prevent SSE, i.e., ride the shudders.

To help yourself focus you can also simultaneously jam your finger, or ask O to jam hers, hard into your perineum.

Beware, though, that riding the shudders more than twice in a session may push you too far the other way and make you lose your erection altogether.

The Sexual Stillpoint

To enable both you and O (when appropriate) to enter the sexual nirvana realm, you have to find the Sexual Stillpoint, which occurs of itself when the sexual energy has built to optimum level during the dance and you are able to lie completely still with boy-O's penis inside O-girl.

This, however, is not an inert stillness, but an active one. Both Os are charged to the maximum possible without actually coming. Boy-O's penis is throbbing/pulsating and O-girl's vaginal walls are contracting and relaxing around O's penis rhythmically in time with the penis's pulsating.

Only the slightest movement is occasionally necessary to maintain momentum of the sexual charge.

It is in this space that your mutual inner-alchemical experiments are conducted.

It is important anyway to alternate movement with rest. There is no advantage gained from constantly pounding away like an industrial, mechanized jackhammer.

Once you've found it, feel free to come in and out of the Sexual Stillpoint for moments of inner refreshment any time you like and as often as you (both) wish.

Full-power pumping

There are times when the Tao of the dance requires you and O to pump away with full power and at maximum speed for a considerable length of time. This is like an orchestra playing a fast and furious crescendo for longer than the musicians might have expected because the conductor's got one on that day. It requires great stamina to do this, especially if you strain. The key to full-power pumping is to breathe deeply, slowly, and softly while completely relaxing the entire body, especially the lower back, the back of the neck, and the belly, and use only the muscle groups necessary to make the movement. It also helps, when lying face-to-face, if the one on top has something to push the soles of his/her feet against, such as a bed frame.

Alternating rhythms

Another factor involved in creating variations in the sexual charge while fucking is to vary the tempo of your thrusts. Sometimes slow, sometimes medium, sometimes fast.

It is a misconception that sex gets more exciting the faster you go. The excitement of speed is superficial. Any stimulation repeated for long enough eventually causes numbness, no matter how good it is.

In any position, using whichever thrusting pattern you like, alternate between slow, medium, and fast thrust tempos.

Do two rounds of any pattern at slow tempo, followed by two rounds at medium tempo. Go back to slow again for a couple of rounds and then do two fast rounds.

Return to slow as your basic walking speed to regroup and regather your energy.

Fucking O in the ass

It is usual to discuss this issue with O beforehand. In fact, this is fast becoming a frequently discussed topic at some of the most fashionable dinner parties in town.

Taking it in the ass is no newfangled fashion thing, however. Though more usually associated with gay men, butt-fucking has been practiced globally for millennia (at least). The French, for example (there they are again), have it as a custom in certain regions, mostly along the eastern borders, upheld by the women to prevent unwanted pregnancies, as do the Irish in some quarters.

Fucking O-girl in the ass is like laying claim to every bit of territory there is, and can be a highly erotic/bestial and scintillating experience for both parties as long as sufficient lubricant is factored into the equation.

It is also essential, in order to preclude what can be excruciating pain for O-girl, to proceed extremely slowly.

It often works best after regular intercourse when O-girl has enjoyed two or three orgasms already and is completely relaxed and has surrendered to the Tao of the dance.

Simply adapt all information regarding entry protocol, thrusting patterns, and the Sexual Stillpoint given above for use during vaginal intercourse. Boy-O needs to be particularly sensitive, perceptive, and alert to the slightest signal from O-girl to indicate either pleasure or pain.

It also helps to jolly up the party if O-girl has managed to empty her bowels, either naturally or by taking an enema prior to the session, to preclude unwelcome mess.

It is also best, after enjoying (or even hating) a round of anal intercourse, for boy-O to either wash his penis carefully and/or change condoms (where applicable) before inserting his penis into O-girl's vagina or mouth, in order to avoid spreading harmful bacteria unnecessarily.

Grinding
this is applicable to both vaginal and anal penetration.

To vary the stimulus of your thrusts, as well as to employ different thrust patterns and tempo changes, you can also grind, as in moving your hips in a circular pattern so that the penis is circling around the vagina as opposed to thrusting in and out.

Grind eighteen times counterclockwise and eighteen clockwise.

Combine grinding with thrusting, circling while simultaneously thrusting in and out, if you can get your head/hips around it.

Augmenting coital stimulation with hand/foot/mouth action

Although there are moments when it is appropriate to fuck with no hands, as in having your pelvis as the only point of contact with O, it is more usually appropriate to supplement and support the pelvic action by using your hands, feet, lips, and tongue to stroke, squeeze, caress, scratch, pinch, tickle, lick, kiss, bite, and/or French kiss O simultaneously, in order to enhance the sexual consciousness connection between you, and to increase the mutual exchange of sexual love.

While engaged in intercourse, lying front to front, for example, if you feel the action's getting too ethereal for your liking, grab O's ass, or reach around and touch O's genitals while he/she engages in his/her intense interchange of Yin and Yang with yours. This has the effect of drawing O's consciousness and your own downward to the lower Tan Tien region, and tends to generate a few more degrees of healthy bestiality.

If, on the other hand, you feel the action's getting too bestial, spend some time doing zygomatic (cheek) kisses, for example, to draw energy away from the genitals and lower Tan Tien up into the brain and upper Tan Tien and thus transform it into the more ethereal pure sexual intelligence (PSI).

Refer to the various "techniques" in this handbook to remind yourself of some of the possible auxiliary hand, foot, and mouth actions that can be used to augment your fucking.

Don't be shy about using your feet at any time to massage and caress O's feet, lower legs, or whichever of O's body parts are to hand (foot). To do this, it is always best to check first that you remembered to remove your shoes and socks before beginning.

Transcendental aspect

The above depicted scenes of debauchery, frolicking, and bonking are all examples of the external aspects of Taoist sex. However, these are just the forms through which you and O can experience the internal, transcendental aspects, wherein you literally transcend the limitations of physical form, to float together (or alone) in the formless realm of sexual nirvana and experience an (eternal) moment of enlightenment (whatever the fuck that is). [See *Sexual nirvana*, p. 67.]

To actualize this requires that you maintain yourself in the mindful/meditative state throughout the sexual dance, using your breath as the psychological lever to keep the door to your inner realms open. [See *Breathing*, p. 112.]

The inner realm is organized around your Three Tan Tiens [See *The Three Tan Tiens*, p. 46], which together comprise your psycho-spiritual center, i.e., the core structure of your Immortal Spirit Body. Keep a thought on your three Tan Tiens (TTTs) at all times during the proceedings.

From the start to the finish of the dance, observe serenely from the upper Tan Tien in the center of your brain, as desire rises and falls from the lower Tan Tien in your belly/loins. Observe serenely as passion mounts and dismounts in the middle Tan Tien in the center of your chest.

Observe serenely, but not clinically, feeling the passion, feeling the desire, but not getting lost in it, i.e., not falling off your log, but remaining centered in your core.

You observe yourself passionately French-kissing O, you feel the passion, you love the passion, you see yourself swimming in it for eternity (with O), *and* you observe yourself doing/feeling/thinking all of it. This doesn't split you in two. To the contrary, it splits you in one.

While observing the rise and fall of passion/desire, you will notice a Yin-Yanging effect. The energy rises. The energy falls. This natural alternation must be followed but not interfered with. In other words, when you feel the intensity of the sexual charge diminish, relax and allow it to do so. Don't panic, simply breathe and wait for the next upturn. Stop and drink a cup of tea together, go watch a movie or whatever, and resume the dance later once the charge has had a chance to build up again.

You might also consider the possibility of extending and maintaining this state of mindfulness permanently, whatever you're doing, till you die (if you're serious about the enlightenment thing, that is).

Connecting your Three (Six) Tan Tiens
that sounds painful.

It's not (trust me—I'm a barefoot doctor).

While fucking face-to-face, mouth kissing mouth, tongue touching tongue, chest pressed to chest, belly merged with belly, visualize a psychic energy channel running from the center of your brain, through your (touching) tongues, into the center of O's brain. You breathe out, O breathes in. As you breathe out, visualize a stream of white light passing along the channel from your brain into O's. Simultaneously, O is breathing in and sucking the light into center brain. O then breathes out, passing the light back to you, while you breathe in to receive it.

Repeat this cycle nine times, then stop, be still, and feel your upper Tan Tiens merge into one.

Jiggle your sexual organs around a bit to keep the sexual charge/boy-O's dick up.

Now visualize a similar channel running from deep inside the center of your chest, through the middle of your breastbone, through the middle of O's breastbone, deep into the center of O's chest.

You breathe out. O breathes in. As you do so, visualize the transmission of a stream of deep crimson light through the channel into O. O receives this by breathing in. You then inhale and receive the light back. Complete nine cycles, then be still together and feel your middle Tan Tiens merge into one.

Do some more genital jiggling in your own special way.

Now visualize a psychic tube running from deep inside the center of your lower abdomen, through a point one inch or so below your navel, through a point one inch or so below O's navel, ending up deep inside the center of O's belly.

As you exhale, visualize golden light streaming through the tube from your lower Tan Tien into O's, while O inhales to receive it. As you inhale, receive the light back in while O exhales to send it. Repeat nine cycles, rest for a moment, and feel your lower Tan Tiens merge into one (joined at the hip).

More genital jiggling.

Then, as you breathe out, visualize/feel the three shades of light moving through their three respective tubes at once, hitting all three of O's Tan Tiens at the same time, while O inhales to receive. As you breathe in, feel the light hitting all three of your Tan Tiens at once, while O exhales to send it. Repeat this cycle nine times, then rest together in the Sexual Stillpoint, feeling your six Tan Tiens merged into one shared core.

This activates the temporary merging of the cores of your two Spirit Bodies into one.

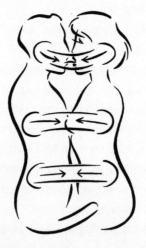

Whooshing the Chi

This is to temporarily bind your Spirit Body with O's, so that you don't get lost or separated while floating together in the formless realm of sexual nirvana.

It also has the effect of protecting each of you from each other's negative chi, which will otherwise invade and infiltrate.

In addition, it has a strong synergistic effect on your positive chi and leaves you feeling like a thousand enlightened beings who've been meditating on a mountaintop together for three days, all merged into one huge energized shape, i.e., you. In other words, it is extremely good for your health in every way.

For this reason it is best not to Whoosh the Chi with an O who's sick, or whose energy is negative, unless you're either feeling excessively strong and possessed of an overabundance of positive chi, or wish to be drained and weakened for spiritually masochistic reasons of your own.

To save overly complex explanations, refer to Scoopin' the Loop before attempting this.

Whooshing the Chi is carried out in two phases: Whooshing the Chi One and Whooshing the Chi Two.

Whooshing the Chi One is performed while fucking in front-to-front mode, preferably during the Sexual Stillpoint just after connecting your respective Tan Tiens. It can be done face-to-face, chest to chest, and belly to belly, or merely belly to belly.

Visualize the internal energy loop running up the back of your spine, over your brain, and down the front of your spine into your perineum. Visualize O's same energy loop. O does likewise. Be aware that your two internal loops are connected at the genitals.

Synchronize your breathing with O's so that you're both breathing in and out at the same time.

As you inhale, visualize that you're pulling in O's sexual energy through your genitals. Feel it ascending the loop, streaming over the top of your head and down into the back of your throat. As you breathe out, visualize it streaming down the front section of the loop into your perineum and genitals, ready to be sucked in by O as O inhales.

O does likewise (simultaneously).

In other words, as you and O breathe in simultaneously, you're sucking each other's chi into your respective internal energy loops, Scoopin' the Loop with it and sending it back again.

Complete nine cycles of this, augmenting it with a lesser Big Squeeze each time you inhale, if you want, then rest together in the oneness of Tan Tien, genitally jiggling to maintain the sexual charge as required.

For Whooshing the Chi Two, you need to be fucking O face-to-face, mouth to mouth, tongue to tongue, center chest to center chest and belly to belly, preferably during the Sexual Stillpoint.

As with Whooshing One, synchronize your breathing with O's so that you're both breathing in and out at the same time.

Breathe O's chi in through your genitals, up the back sector of your loop, and over your brain into your tongue.

O does likewise.

Now breathe the chi out through your tongue into O's tongue and down the front sector of O's loop to O's perineum and genitals.

O does likewise.

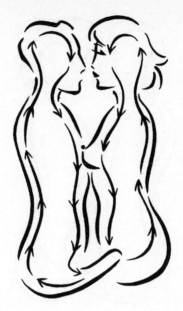

You then breathe the chi in through each other's genitals and start the cycle again.

Complete nine cycles, then (both of you) do the Big Squeeze, pop through the veil (you'll see what I mean when you get there—maybe/probably), and chill together in the spiritual wonderland of sexual nirvana (because there's nothing much else to do around there). [See *Sexual nirvana*, p. 67.]

If, at this point, boy-O decides to forgo a good squirt and shudder, he will be energized for days after, as will O-girl, who will feel this no matter how many times she's managed to orgasm during the session, in fact the more the merrier.

If, on the other hand, boy-O decides to go for the easy/familiar option, i.e., ejaculation, he will have a most refined explosion, then roll over and start snoring (probably).

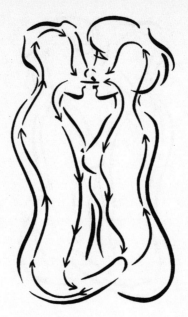

Don't get too holy/earnest/reverent/serious about this sexual nirvana business, however, for as with most things Taoist, no matter how earth-movingly effective they are, they're only really intended as a bit of a laugh (to distract us while we hang around waiting to die, lest ye forget).

Effective postorgasmic phase management

The big bang comes and whams you both out of your skins. As you lie there panting, but ideally breathing deeply, in the raw exposed state of naked spirit, still (ideally) in touch with your three/six Tan Tiens, you start to feel yourselves coming back into your respective bodies.

As you come back into your body, your local mind starts getting busy again. That was nice. How long have I got? What's the time? Wow, that wasn't as long as I thought it was. Shit, I've got to get up and phone Toloto . . ." etc., etc., and you begin to feel progressively separate from O.

Don't feel treacherous about this. O is possibly/probably doing likewise.

Simply observe yourself in transition from one state to another, serenely, without judgment. I mean, hell, we've all got agendas.

However, respect for the fact that you've just shared a moment of sublime oneness with a living manifestation of the Tao itself, i.e., O, must be consciously maintained, as well as sensitivity to the raw open state you and O are in.

As you come back into your body, back into local reality, release the energy strings slowly, as you'd replace a Ming Dynasty vase on the table: carefully.

Removal of the penis at a mutually suitable moment (paying attention to condom integrity where appropriate), and subsequent rearrangement of bodily positions, must be conducted likewise: slowly, carefully, tenderly, and sensitively. It's not like taking a piss, shaking your dick a couple of times, and zipping your fly up (boy-O). As every good warrior knows, you leave as you entered: respectfully.

Stay conscious. Don't pass out. Allowing the energy connection, i.e., love, to continue flowing between you and O, let yourself relax into that delicious postorgasmic near theta state of deep meditation you know and love so well.

And don't talk. Don't ask, "How was I?" Don't even go, "Wow, that was great," or indulge in any other such post–big bang inanities, other than possibly, "I love you," but then only if you have to so much you'll burst otherwise.

Simply be silent and let the spirits/angels/realizations come to you.

However, as being silent at this stage requires mutual cooperation, do not be afraid to give voice to the sound, "Ssshhhh," in patient, loving, quasiconspiratorial tones when necessary, and/or to negotiate postorgasmic silences in advance.

Only when you are instinctively sure that you've returned completely to your local self and that O has done likewise without any stray bits of spirit or errant chi caught among the bedclothes, is it advisable to make your excuses and take your gracious leave, i.e., go and have that piss or whatever.

THEPAYOFF
(postorgasmic blatherings)

What about
sexual problems?
don't talk to me about sexual problems.

But what if I've got one?

Everybody's got one (at least). How could it be otherwise? We're living in a lunatic asylum, ever on the brink of mutual destruction, hormones in the water, radiation and cross-genes in the food, pollution in the air, disease in the bodily fluids, more and more information assailing our senses through more and more media, faster and faster every month/week/day/hour/minute/second. We've got this magazine telling us: be this, think that, do that, feel that; another telling us the opposite; TV programs telling us not very much at all; and now we even have to contend with books like this.

What do you expect? Of course all this stress is going to show up where we're most sensitive. But don't let your sexual problems defeat you, sexually or any other way.

You may have been raped, abused, assaulted, married to a maniac, left by every lover, or molested by a family member.

You may be anatomically deficient, too fat, too thin, too ill, too tired, riddled with complexes, neurotic, or just painfully shy.

You may be perverted, hooked on pornography, addicted to pain (giving and/or receiving), addicted to sex, addicted to falling in love, addicted to masturbation, addicted to being tied up, addicted to drugs, or just plain lazy.

You may be impotent, frigid, obsessed, terrified of condoms, stuck in a rut, unable to settle down, unable to come, or unable to stop yourself from coming.

You may be too small. You may be too big. Hell, you may even be too ugly.

Nobody's perfect (anyway).

But don't let that stop you from exploring all the mad stuff in this handbook, because if you do explore, you may find something rubs off and burns a little hole in your self-limiting patterns.

Don't let self-pity, fear, shame, or guilt stop you from exploring or enjoying sex.

Don't let your features deter you from making friends with people you fancy. You may not think you're the prettiest girl/handsomest boy at the ball, but don't let that stop you from dancing.

Don't let your moral code lead you up a blind alley.

Don't let your lack of morals make you forget who you really are.

Don't identify with your "problem." Identify with the positive aspect, i.e., the solution.

But do excuse me for generalizing so universally and presenting a remedy so glibly. However, it is essential to remember that you create your own experience of reality. That means that from here on in you can create it beautiful or ugly. That's entirely up to you.

Work with what you have, however deficient you may be or feel you are in various ways. Celebrate the sexuality of who you are (right now); don't waste valuable sexual time mourning the fact you're not somebody else.

People love you for your heart and soul. So open your heart and let your soul sing through, and there is nothing you want that won't come to you (within reason).

There, are you feeling better now, dear?

Rape

Every good warrior knows that if you violate another person's space (in any way), according to the immutable law of cause and effect, your own space will later be violated three times worse.

If you've been the victim of a rape, don't lose your faith in humanity/men or yourself. Have the faith to forgive yourself for being there and the faith to believe that whatever occurs in your life does so to ultimately enrich you.

Practice Scoopin' the Loop to cleanse your energy every day for days on end, as well as the Big Squeeze on a regular basis to join yourself back up again. Meditate on harmonizing your TTTs and let this become the backbone of your psychic structure.

If you have raped or are considering doing so in the future, practice the Big Squeeze every hour on the hour for three weeks. This will shift your sexual energy upward and give you a glimpse of what it is to be free of this compulsion, and how it can be sublimated into something more socially productive.

If you think you may have psychopathic tendencies that might lead you to rape someone without realizing what you're doing, meditate endlessly on harmonizing your TTTs, in order to link you together with yourself.

Complexes
everyone has them.

Drop them. That is, drop concerning yourself about them. Carry on regardless of them.

Just say, "Hello, Complex(es), how are you? We're going to have sex with O now, *won't* that be fun!" and take Complex to bed with you.

There's no point trying to banish Complex from the boudoir. Like a spoiled adolescent, that will only make Complex try and fuck you up even more.

If you feel unshapely or awkward as you walk naked across the floor, do so with the fullness of yourself, and let that be sexy. Don't walk across the room pretending to you and/or O that you're actually somebody else.

Be open about your Complex(es). Don't be shy about them.

Just be yourself and let that be good enough. And if that isn't good enough for O, it's not good enough, and O will probably go. And then you'll say, "Darn that barefoot doctor and his crazy handbook, I knew I should have wrapped myself in a blanket [before I walked across the room]."

Frigidity

As in you find it impossible to warm your sexual fires up enough to want sex with O. It doesn't mean you're a freak. It happens all the time. [For male frigidity, see *Impotence*, p. 211.] Practice the Big Squeeze on a daily basis. Masturbate tenderly, with or without fantasy, using oils or lubrication on a regular basis, with the attitude of conducting a form of self-therapy. Talk freely about your mindset apropos sex and your resistance to it, preferably to a professional listener/therapist/counselor. Take up tai chi to stimulate your sexual fire, pay regular visits to an acupuncturist/healer/barefoot doctor to join your energy field back up, and a homeopath to come at it from a different angle.

Vaginismus

When your vagina won't open at all, practice the Big Squeeze once an hour, for days on end. Pay regular visits to a craniosacral therapist, acupuncturist, and homeopath. Have someone you trust spend a regular hour with a finger, lubricated and gently inserted in your vagina, starting with their little finger and gradually working up to their forefinger. This is done with four ounces, without trying to open the vagina. Simply wait patiently while it regains its trust in the world and begins to open slowly around the finger. Once this is easy, move on to bigger things (to insert).

Don't give up, however, till you die. I've seen so many cases clear up that I think you'd be unwise to abandon your vagina at this stage of the game.

Impotence

As in being powerless to manifest an adequate movement of blood into the small blood vessels of your penis for a long enough space of time to fuck somebody.

Prostate gland damage notwithstanding, impotence can usually be effectively remedied by natural methods.

Impotence arises, or rather, occurs, when your kidney fire is deficient. This can be treated with Chinese herbs and acupuncture. Taking up the daily practice of chi kung (pronounced ji gung) and/or tai chi (pronounced tie chee) is also efficacious in reigniting/stoking the flames.

Additionally, practice the Big Squeeze hourly on a daily basis during the summer months, half-hourly in the winter, till you die, as this strengthens the prostate, and practice Scoopin' the Loop every day to join your brain up with your dick (properly).

And if that doesn't work, take Viagra. [See *Warning and disclaimer*, p. 3.]

Nervous willy

Little Willy was scared of the big dark forest. His parents had told him there was a deep cave there with a horrible monster living in it, and that if anyone roamed there at night, the horrible monster would eat him/her.

They only told him this to stop his running off into the forest alone and getting lost. But being small, he believed them.

However, Willy was curious, so one day he plucked up all his courage, girded his loins, puffed up his chest, and stood up as tall as he could, so that he really looked quite big.

Boldly, he strode up to the forest's edge and peered into the darkness. His curiosity growing stronger now, following a hunch, he walked through the thick undergrowth until he got to the cave where the monster lived.

He paused for a moment and drew himself up to his full height. But just as he was about to enter the cave, the monster woke up and roared a terrible roar that resounded for miles around.

Willy froze in fear. As he did, he seemed to wilt, as is often the case when you lose your confidence. He shrank and shrank until he was just tiny little Willy, turned around and ran out of the forest back home in time for tea.

Some storytellers say it happened because he stopped to pull his hood over his head at the entrance and became suddenly flustered. I'd say it just happened. These things do (from time to time).

Sometimes it's because you don't feel safe with the O you're with.

Sometimes it's because you're not meant to be with that O.

Sometimes it's because you've got a lot on your mind.

Always it's because O's Yang is overpowering yours. This might be because O has particularly strong Yang, but is more likely to be because your Yang isn't strong enough.

This can be remedied through daily practice of vigorous martial arts, fast running, cycling, or rock-climbing, i.e., Yang activities.

Hypnotherapy can also be highly effective in talking directly to Willy and negotiating. In addition, spend time visualizing yourself making a successful entrance on a daily basis.

Do the Big Squeeze and Scoopin' the Loop every day to strengthen your Yang and join your intelligence with Willy's.

Don't identify with Nervous Willy. Simply observe yourself in the drama. Nine times out of ten it's just a phase you're going through and will pass before you've had time to say, "Big horrible monster."

Sexually transmitted diseases
(stds)

These are a drag, there's no two ways about it. What's more, they make you ill. If you don't watch out they can even kill you.

There isn't much you can do about it either.

The effects of disease can be lessened by drug cocktails, ointments, and/or various medicines, natural and unnatural. You can learn to view the disease in a positive light for all the invaluable life lessons it brings, but whichever way you shoot the sherbet, Herbert, STDs are a drag.

That is why it is vastly important at this time in our history to use condoms, as these are the *only* way we have at present to control the spread.

There are people alive who go around giving their disease to Os on purpose.

There are people alive who go around giving Os their disease without knowing it.

And you never know who they are. You could be one yourself.

That's why, for all its drawbacks, the condom kicks.

Do not, however, on considering this, employ it as a device to fuel your fears of sex. To be afraid of sex because you're afraid of death is to be afraid of life itself. And to indulge in that for long is unwise, as you only get to do it once (in your present form).

To let your fear of STDs prevent you from enjoying sex is like not breathing because the air's polluted. You don't do that, you keep breathing till the last drop of oxygen's been used up. It's the same with sex. That's how humans are.

Unwanted pregnancy

You didn't use a condom. You didn't take the pill. No cap. No coil. No coitus interruptus. No awareness of when you're/she's ovulating. You/she got pregnant when you didn't want to. What did you expect?

Moral issues and miscarriage wishes aside, your choice now is between a minimum eighteen-year commitment to bringing up a child in an expensive, mad, mad world, tied for as long, however directly or indirectly, to O; growing the baby inside you to full term, then giving it up for adoption; or aborting it before it has time to realize what's going on.

This is not an enviable predicament in which to find yourself. Any of your three choices can lead to overwhelming consequences for everyone involved.

And there's no way around that with any new-age nonsense. It's a horrible place to be.

To prevent this, use birth control. And that's it.

Sudden Surprise
Ejaculation Syndrome
(sses)

Regardless of any psycho-emotional causes, this arises (literally) when boy-O's Yin is deficient. Specifically the Yin of his kidneys. That's why it happens more when you're tired or ill.

Kidney Yin deficiency can be treated effectively with acupuncture and Chinese herbs.

It is helpful to make a conscious outcome choice at the start of any sexual proceedings with O.

Do I want to come as soon as I feel like it?

Do I want to come with O?

Do I want to come after O's already come once or twice?

Do I want to come at all?

Decide on one option clearly, well before penetration begins. Then say to yourself, "That is my choice."

Remaining mindful, as per earlier instructions in this book, observe yourself uninterruptedly, breathing slowly and deeply, making ample use of the Big Squeeze as often as you can, and otherwise occupying yourself with the head fuck of following the "techniques," resorting as often as necessary to pulling back to the entrance and remaining perfectly still and even riding the shudders if you've the nerve. It should be possible for you to catch the goblin that usually triggers SSES when you're not looking, before the little bastard has time to pull the switch. Then again, maybe it won't be.

Let's face it, sometimes that O-girl is just too damn sexy for you, boy-O.

Inability to orgasm

You have to differentiate here between the inability to come while
having sex with an O, and the inability to come at all.

If it's the former, but you find it perfectly simple and straightforward to come when you masturbate, then masturbate when
you're having sex with O. (And/or teach O how to do it for you.)

If it's the latter and you don't even know how to make yourself
come, *then* you've got a problem.

This problem can be addressed, however, by an experienced sex
therapist, hooker, acupuncturist, hypnotherapist, jumping out of a
second-floor window and subsequently having a revelatory experience in the hospital, or simply giving up and becoming permanently celibate.

The above suggestion of jumping from a window may sound extreme and far-fetched. While extreme it is, far-fetched it isn't. This
actually happened to a girl I know, and she's been coming like a
stormtrooper ever since. It was the shock to her system that broke
the spell and woke her up to who she really was, a fully functioning
(if broken-boned) sexual being. [See *Warning and disclaimer*, p. 3.]

The Big Squeeze, practiced on a daily basis alongside occasional
application by a willing O of Toe in the Hole, may also do wonders. [See *Toe in the Hole*, p. 154.]

Sadomasochism,
bondage, marriage,
and other perversions

Restricting your spirit, through pain, inflicted or received, the
application of ropes, pulleys, handcuffs, leather/rubber straps and
apparel, or legal channels, i.e., subjugating your own will in sub-

mission to the will of another, may well be something you wish to spend your time here (on earth) doing.

The Wayward Taoist belief, however, is that it is preferable to afford yourself and any/every O with whom you consort, the utmost freedom possible at all times. This freedom includes freedom from pain inflicted by you, or vice versa, whether it be physical, emotional, psychological, or a combination of all three. That includes the psychological, emotional, and sometimes physical pain of being legally obliged to permit an O to live out their real-time story line over your own, even when you expressly don't want them to and/or indeed have an extreme aversion to their doing so.

Not to say there's anything wrong with marriage. I did eleven years myself, spread over two terms. I mean, it's something you do, isn't it? For the romance of joining the clichéd throngs and asking, "Will you marry me?" For the dress. For the ceremony. For that primal moment of carrying her/being carried by him over the threshold. For that first fuck as Mr. and Mrs. For the children you have or will have. For the money. For an escape from a boring life. For a sense of belonging. For the house. For the children. For the fear of change. For the alimony. For the simple reason that you were stupid and fell off your rocker at the wrong moment. For the immigration papers. For status. For playing Mommies and Daddies (i.e., yours). For the reason that you are both mature adults, who, not being caught up in any romantic Cole Porter claptrap, have decided, calmly, intelligently, logically, and clearheadedly to legally bind yourselves with society as your witness, to stay faithful, loyal, and loving to the other person exclusively, till one of you dies, *or* you get divorced.

However, the trance of this extreme form of bondage is so strongly inculcated into our very blueprints that even though the original socioeconomic causes for doing it are no longer in any way valid (in so-called modern culture), we all of us, including silly barefoot doctors, can fall prey at any time. (So beware.)

Prostitution

In an ideal Wayward world, professional prostitutes would get the respect they deserve for saving more marriages than all the other caring professions put together.

They would be legally recognized and regulated by a governing body, say the National Institute of Chartered Prostitutes, or its foreign equivalent.

They would be trained in the arts of sexology, joke-telling, self-defense (to deal with physically abusive customers), and general hostess/host skills, much like the geisha girls/boys of old.

They would eschew the use of drugs and would be trained in metaphysics (so as not to lose their souls during working hours) and how to avoid crack, smack, and/or alcohol addiction, and they would be regularly screened for infectious diseases.

As it is, however, they are marginalized to the outer edges of society, mostly outside the protection of the law. If one gets killed by a vicious pimp, the chances are no one, including the law, will care, because they're "only hookers."

Not that I'm saying that girls/boys work for altruistic, selfless reasons. Who does, except the odd Mother Teresa or two? But for the risks they take and the actual therapeutic good they do, it would seem just that their status in society should be elevated to at least that of, say, stockbrokers or real estate agents, who, though they number some fine chaps among their ranks, do not actually contribute nearly as much to society in real-time as hookers.

As it is, hookers have a fairly hard time of it. Not just the girls/boys who work the streets, but also the top-class hookers, who, with the odd exception, invariably turn to crack, smack, alcohol, and/or worse, to numb the existential pain of renting out their soul/hole.

Though I haven't used the services of a prostitute since I was a schoolboy doing it for a lark (and of course a cheap fuck) with my friends, I have, over the years, made the acquaintance, through my work, of some very high-class hookers as well as the (very) odd madam, which is how I developed an empathy. It made me look at the prostitute within me. And by contrast to many nonworking girls, they are refreshingly honest about their motivations.

If you find yourself into, or sliding into, this line of work, be aware that once in, it becomes absurdly difficult to get out, mostly on account of the money, of course, but also because of the twilight-zone lifestyle, from which it is often impossible to readjust. If, however, you are committed to this path, practice Scoopin' the Loop and Three Tan Tiens awareness to help maintain the integrity of your Spirit Body and reinforce your protective energy field.

If you have or are contemplating using the services of a hooker, do so with respect, and remember that all women are expressions of the universal female archetype, the Great Mother, and must be honored as such, no matter how they earn their money. (For boy hookers, substitute men for women, male archetype for female, and Great Scott for Great Mother.)

Threesomes/fivesomes/ sevensomes/orgies

Trios can certainly be fun, for a short while at least, but generally turn out to prove right the dictum that three's a crowd.

Ideally, threesomes should be an opportunity for you to express your love in stereo. But this is rarely the case. For when the drugs wear off and/or the lust is spent, what the fuck are you going to do with two people in your bed? It's often hard enough trying to get to sleep with one person snoring next to you, let alone two. Not to mention all that awkward giggling and lining up to use the bathroom afterward.

Nevertheless, if ever presented with the opportunity to make love with two Os at once, and you find the gender combination and general attributes on display to your liking, it is the strong recommendation of this handbook that you give it a go. If only for the theater.

In actual fact, from a boy-O's perspective, if you can arrange it, and it's a large if, it works far better to be with six women at once than just two: one on one hand, one on the other, one on one foot, one on the other, one sitting on your dick, and one sitting on your face. At least that way it keeps your mind from wandering or getting caught up in vying for someone's attention.

For O-girls, the equivalent, though a little unfair, is to have only four men: one to fuck you conventionally, one to fuck you in the ass, one to put his dick in your mouth and/or massage and caress you, and one to do the shopping and cleaning. However, the danger here is of your boudoir smelling like the men's changing room at the health club, and the conversation can probably get a bit stiff at times, or so I'm told.

Obviously these two scenarios are pretty straightforward, because I'm a bit of a prude, and I'm sure you've come across far more bizarre combinations on your travels. Whichever combination you may find yourself involved with in the future, however, it is important to remember, if beset by feelings of existential or sexual disorientation during any of the proceedings, that the reason you come together is to share love, and if you can do that effectively, with or without drugs or alcohol, with just one other person, let alone two, four, or six, you're doing well.

Keep your heart open to love whomever you're with, scoop a lot of loop to protect you from negative chi, and remain centered in your TTTs throughout to retain some sense of identity.

Sex parties

How boring these events are. Even public libraries carry more of a sexual charge in the air.

When you turn sex into an organized spectator/participation sport, it tends to remove the erotic element. There's nothing very sexy about watching loads of odd-shaped women squeezed into clichéd dominatrix uniforms or French maids' outfits, politely leading flabby men in rubber suits around on all fours by rings through their noses, like Mary with her little lamb, or sitting having a chat with an old friend while a leather-clad woman next to you fucks some idiot with a polite cheesy grin on his face. It's more of a turn-on watching people eating at the next table in a restaurant.

Not that there's anything wrong with this kind of exhibitionism, voyeurism, lighthearted s 'n' m, or even fancy dress, but does it actually have anything to do with sex? (Or maybe I've just been to the wrong parties?)

Perversion

Anything you wouldn't do yourself and think is kind of weird is usually referred to as a perversion, and practitioners thereof, perverts or pervs.

However, is there really anything that two people can do together by clear mutual consent, during the sexual dance, however weird, that can objectively be called perverted?

If you feel compelled to piss all over O in the bath for instance, and O is happy about that, is it actually perverted to follow your compulsion through? And if so, by whose standards?

If, on the other hand, you felt that compulsion but O was not in any way desirous of your acting it out, but you went ahead and sprinkled away regardless, that would be perverted. Perverted in the sense that you perverted the inherent, tacit agreement to respect the wishes of one another and not to do any weird shit without the other's full consent.

Like if O wants to sniff your shoes, kiss them, rub up against them, and even clean them for you, sure it's a bit pervy, but what have you got to lose? Just be sure not to let him or her polish your sneakers, because that *would* be perverted.

The problem of incest

This is a problem, not just between brothers and sisters, fathers and daughters, fathers and sons, uncles and nieces, aunties and nephews, grandfathers and granddaughters, but also mothers and sons (I met such a couple only the other day), even mothers and daughters, and though I have never been told firsthand by either party of such misdoings between grandmother and grandson, I'm sure it happens.

Originally, if you believe in such spurious conjecture as mooted in our creation myth, there were just Adam and Eve. So it follows that everyone thereafter, including you and me, was/is committing incest.

Lot, the pillar of salt dude from Sodom and Gomorrah, even admitted in writing to impregnating his own daughter.

But even if you believe in that old Adam and Eve baloney, and thus find justification for acting out your incestuous urges, surely you must agree it's a matter of degree, and that restraint is called for here, if only for the sake of minimizing emotional, psychological, spiritual, sexual, and genetic confusion levels on the planet?

Because that's the one single common denominator I've found among all the (vast) numbers of people I've met/treated, who've been coerced, subtly or otherwise, by older or more powerful family members; into acting out incestuous sex: overwhelming, undermining confusion.

If you are one of these, my heart goes out to you, in the hope that you have/find the courage to accept and forgive yourself and the offending family member, in order that you may be able to join up all the fragments of self again and move on to enjoying blissful, innocent, healthy sex with appropriate Os, and not repeat the pattern with your own offspring. This process can be more easily facilitated by in-depth therapy/counseling and/or healing.

The problem of child abuse

While it's true that every child is born with full sexual awareness, it is usually not until that child has reached at least sixty-two that it has any real sense of who it is, where it stands in the world, and thus has formed some idea of how best to accommodate its primal sexual urges.

If, however, we ruled that sex with anyone below the age of sixty-two was immoral/criminal, not only would there be a dangerous reduction in the number of new people born, it would also be just plain stupid.

So in our lenient wisdom we have arbitrarily defined age limits, usually coinciding with the latter stages of puberty, once the hormones have had time to settle, below which it is illegal/criminal/immoral to have sex.

Obviously, this is nonsense where it involves two fully consenting "underage" lovers, who know what they're doing, or are finding out fast, are clued up about condoms, etc., and who by complete free will find themselves exploring the depths of their love, lust, and passion together. I think that only the most dried-out bore would think that was anything other than the couple's own business. Hell, I had two of the most memorable fucks of my life before I was fourteen. How about you?

That notwithstanding, when a so-called adult manipulates a child/underage adolescent into acting out the sexual urge, even if that urge is apparently mutual, he/she is violating boundaries which haven't yet had time to form properly, and it is like forcing a baby to walk before its legs are sufficiently developed, i.e., it fucks them up for life.

And I'm not talking about a sixteen- or seventeen-year-old doing it with a fifteen-year-old, I'm talking about grown men (and women) doing it with children who subsequently spend the rest of their lives sorting out/living with the damage.

And, yes, I'm angry (about it). If you spent time talking with a beautiful, sane woman of thirty-nine, who still can't sleep at night sometimes because of the painful memory of the things a fully grown man coerced her into doing with him between the ages of seven and eleven, not to mention all the countless other stories; if you'd witnessed the tortured, haunted look on her face, you'd probably be angry too.

I myself at the beautiful, blond, curly-haired, innocent age of three, allowed *myself* to be manipulated on more than one occasion, albeit extremely dextrously and sensually, by my nanny, who was thirty at the time, into going down on her to perform cunnilingus.

Fortunately, these forays into the deep dark forest of Nanny Catherine's female mystery did nothing to dampen my ardor for this magnificent "sport." Quite the contrary. It did, however, instigate an innate confusion about personal boundaries, so that even with the help of some of the greatest psychotherapists on the planet, including the late R. D. Laing and Frank B. Kramer, I still have a problem saying "no" to beautiful women sometimes, especially ones called Catherine. (Nice problem, though.) Nanny, by the way, ended up in a loony bin, not because of that, she was nuts anyway, and is probably dead by now, bless her.

Sex toys

Sex toys are fun. All toys are fun. Till the batteries run out. Or you get bored, which you usually do if you play with them too much. Toys usually won't do it for you like the real thing does, unless the real thing you're doing isn't so hot or you've got a damn good toy.

However, toys are helpful in redressing the balance between two lovers of widely differing libido levels, as in O-girl wants/needs/requires far more attention from hard phallic objects than boy-O can naturally muster. For example, if fit young O-girl's boy-O is a bit of an old boy-O, tired boy-O, sick boy-O, or anatomically challenged boy-O, and can't get it up so often these days, and refuses, on account of good common sense and general sanity, to go without Viagra, the judicious use of an efficient vibrator can do wonders, especially when augmented by oral and manual stimulatory activities.

Not to mention the benefits when you're on your own with a lazy wrist.

Lubricants

Use them liberally to avoid genital/anal soreness. Obviously it is preferable, in most instances, to use natural lubricants composed of vaginal fluid and saliva, but where these are not readily available in sufficient abundance, always have access to a handy pot of natural coconut oil or lubricating jelly. But remember to use only water-based lubricants with condoms, to prevent rubber rot.

Aphrodisiacs

Although there are certain recognized chemicals, herbs, aromas, and tastes which can produce a temporary increase in libido levels, one O's meat is another O's poison.

While oysters, for instance, may render one O quite fruity, they may make another O run to the bathroom and throw up. Ylang-ylang may tease the desires of one O but leave another running for the fresh air spray. Swallowing GHB may return one boy-O to his natural animal state while turning another psychotic.

The only true aphrodisiac is the erotic dialogue (verbal and/or otherwise) that occurs naturally, of itself, when the time, place, dynamics, context, and chemistry are just right. This is so, regardless of whether you're eating oysters or Spam, whether you've doused yourself in ylang-ylang or (heaven forbid) Chanel No. 5.

The aphrodisiac effect of such an erotic moment arises through providence, not contrivance. If you feel the need to contrive in this manner, it's time to look closely at your insecurities and devise a plan to minimize their effect on your behavioral repertoire with the help of a competent therapist.

Alcohol and sex

Generally good for girls. Bad for boys.

(Most) girls will do almost anything when they're smashed. (Most) boys just fall asleep and snore.

From the male perspective, however, sex with a woman who's off her trolley on booze tends to be unsatisfying on a deeper level.

On the other hand, a moderate amount of fine wine and/or champagne (or tequila/vodka or whatever) may be helpful to both boy-Os and O-girls to loosen the grip of the odd inhibition here and there at certain times, but should not be relied upon (in any way) as a long-term animal-nature lubricant.

Drugs and sex

This depends on the drug, who's taking it (with whom), and under what circumstances.

(I'm neither advocating, nor advising you to eschew, the use of the following list of drugs, nor any other of the myriad concoctions available that do not appear on the list, though I would say it's always better for your psychic, spiritual, emotional, and physical health to take your experiences in a naturally induced state of mind whenever possible/plausible.)

Cannabis tends to make you more sensitive to what's going on, but can easily increase feelings of insecurity and paranoia at precisely the wrong moments.

Cocaine tends to enhance sexual satisfaction among women (in the short term), but sometimes, though not always, tends to make willies shrivel.

Acid can take you to either extreme. It has the potential to turn your sexual dance into an extremely elegant ballet performed by angels, or an extremely macabre ball performed by demons and ghouls. Alternatively, it can leave you completely nonplussed and confused about what a willy's used for and where to put it (on both sides).

MDMA can synthesize pleasure of such intensity that your heart wants to burst all over O, but like cocaine can just as easily make you shrivel.

Ketamine tends to detach you so much from any connection with your physical form, you don't even know where your private parts are, let alone what to do with them.

Heroin's heroin.

And I'm bored talking about drugs now, save to say that a sexual love scenario based on you and O taking drugs (of any sort) will only ever go as deep as the drugs and will not truly touch your soul. (Though I'm quite happy to be proven wrong.)

The problem of sexual possessiveness

This isn't just a problem, it's a monster. People kill on account of it. People trap one another in the most sinister webs of emotional blackmail and psychologically coercive tactics because of it. People drive themselves half-crazy/full-crazy on its account.

And it's a complete illusion. True, it's an illusion that people expend inordinate amounts of energy upholding, but an illusion nevertheless.

You don't possess anyone. You don't even possess yourself. And if you don't believe me, wait till the reaper comes along and then tell me what you possess. So to even begin to think about possessing an O is blatant absurdity.

Drop it. Let things be. If O finds someone else to play with in the playground, let O go. If O's meant to return, O will.

Of course you'll feel jealous. But jealousy's only jealousy. Acknowledge its presence when beset by such an attack, accept it graciously, don't deny it, even admit it to those concerned and you may find it loosens its horrible grip on your thoughts and your guts. Or you may find it doesn't, in which case you'll just have to remain in the blind-animal-running-around-a-maze state for a while longer.

Don't cling to your idea of what's your territory. Be fluid about it and trust that if your O should go, there's an even better one for you (for now) waiting just in the wings. Always trust that (or you may go nuts).

Pornography as a stimulant

Watching a porno movie or looking at porno mags with O can be just the stimulant you both need to kick-start the action. The Japanese had their erotic pillow books. The Chinese had their erotic art. We've got Internet porno sites, porno mags, and movies. So what?

However, if you happen to be a lonesome boy-O using this kind of visual stimulus, or telephone sex lines for that matter, in order to inspire you during a masturbation session, be sure to have a box of tissues handy.

Cozy/lazy vs. sexy

There comes a time in most sexual love scenarios, especially those of a domestic nature, when sexy gets insidiously replaced by cozy, i.e., lazy.

As you both lie there enjoying your cozy cuddles, it can be hard/embarrassing/too strenuous to transcend the state of cozy in order to attain to the state of erotic excitement.

This is especially so when you're both tired, the kids are screaming/demanding, your mind is trapped in agenda reality, or you just don't feel sexy.

It's true, anyone'll tell you, though the love may be strong and the cuddles sublime, sex in long-term "relationships" can get extremely dull. It's a fact.

But what to do about it?

Talk about it. Go and see a couples' counselor. Get into massaging each other. Make a special effort once a week (flowers, dinner, candles, perfume, hairdos, soft music on the stereo, the sheets turned back, etc.). Try some of the weirder stuff in this handbook. Have an affair. Run off with the gardener. Run off with your next-door neighbor. Become celibate. I mean, I don't know. What are you asking me for?

What I *do* know, however, is, if at all possible, avoid limiting O with your own limited beliefs and projections. Don't limit O to being the cozy-cuddles Mommy/Daddy figure. See O's potential to be the fiery lover you want. You can be sure that she/he could easily be that with/for some other O right now, so let her/him be that for you, by seeing her/him so.

As you see it, so will it be. See O as a frump and that's exactly how O will show up for you. See O as a magnificent sexual being and that's what O will be (in theory). Like I said, I don't know, do I?

It always helps to get dressed up, go out to a swanky do, and show each other off. Flirt a bit with a few people to stir a little jealousy. Step out of your workaday local roles of Mr. and Mrs., Mommy and Daddy, whatever, and let yourselves once again feel the sensation of being the unique individuals who fell in love with each other enough to get yourselves into this mess in the first place.

Using sex as a distraction

Well, it's better than watching television.

Using sex as a form of stress relief

Only effective in the short term, i.e., it just works till you get out of bed, off the kitchen table, out of the telephone booth, or wherever you've just been relieving your stress. Better to take up tai chi and far less sticky in the long run.

The problem of fluctuating libido levels

Everybody's level of sexual energy and therefore sexual interests fluctuate according to time of day, time of month, season, age, health, stamina, climate, diet, drug/alcohol intake, work/financial pressure levels, as well as a host of other unseen factors.

This is natural/normal and not to be fretted over unless you find yourself uncomfortably at either extreme (phobic or manic) for too long, in which case seek the help of a competent acupuncturist, herbalist, naturopath, therapist, and/or whatever.

When, however, you put two people together for any significant space of time, each with his/her own individual patterns of fluctuation, it is bound to make for interesting dialogue from time to time. (At least.)

When your O will not let go, try massage. It often works. There is a particularly good book called *The Tao of Sexual Massage*, which I usually recommend (because I wrote it).

Celibacy

It is essential to give yourself a breather from time to time, to clear out the residue of any distorted energy patterns you may have picked up from Os along the way, and to regroup. (Any good hooker will tell you that.)

Award yourself periods of voluntary celibacy every now and then. Two weeks is adequate for a basic regroup and rebalance session, but you may want to extend this for anywhere up to nine months.

Beyond that and you're going down a different spiritual path altogether, quite outside the scope of this book and the experience of its author. In other words, you're on your own with that one, baby.

Always be prepared

Never leave home without first ensuring that your physical person has been subjected to sufficient standards of hygiene to withstand the scrutiny and gain the approval of any O you might happen to find yourself engaged in the sexual love dance with that day. And always have (at least) one condom sequestered conveniently about your person.

Because you never know whom you're going to meet, or when, and it would be a damn shame to blow it because you were too smelly and unprepared.

Using sex as a substitute for human warmth

That's fine every now and again, but it might be better/less sticky if you investigate the pleasure of hugging people and cuddling your friends instead.

Sex with strangers vs.
sex with your mate

Well, it happens. Of that there's no denying. And what's more it can be exciting in the short term. No denying that either. It may, however, leave you feeling ashamed, guilty, and confused, and probably force you to lie (even more) to your mate, which further compounds your shame, guilt, and confusion. Then again, it may not.

(You'll do what you do, when you do it, how you do it, and that's all there is to it. Just do it with a condom—for everyone's sake.)

Sex with friends

Better than sex with enemies, isn't it?

The problem of
promiscuity/sex addiction

Promiscuity, like celibacy, is an extreme. Any extreme lifestyle maintained indefinitely is usually bad for your health. Practice Scoopin' the Loop and Whooshing the Chi, as well as the Big Squeeze as often and regularly as you can during sex, as this will spiritualize your encounters, which in itself tends to burn holes in negative patterns. Not that I'm saying there's anything negative about sharing sexual love with many people. Far from it. Just that you may want to look closely at your motivations from time to time. Perhaps you are fundamentally sexually insecure and therefore have a compulsive need to keep proving again (and again) (and again!?) that you are actually good enough. All right, you're good enough. Can we stop now?

Interestingly, dolphins, arguably one of the highest evolved species on the planet (maybe even more evolved than you and I), who are well known for their considerable healing qualities, are so "promiscuous" that they'll fuck anyone, any time, any place, without seeming to display any "moral" qualms about monogamy and other such human trifles.

But if you want to treat it as an addiction, go right ahead.

Pregnancy and sex

Do it. It's good for you. You won't hurt the baby. Do it from behind (after the third month, or at your discretion).

Sex in the nine months or so after pregnancy

Tricky.

Marriage and sex

Awful. (Kidding.)

Divorce and sex

Better. (Not kidding.)

Age differences

One of the most loving, successful, genuinely harmonious, and sexually active long-term "relationships" I know is a boy-O in his early thirties and an O-girl of sixty-nine. They've been together for over ten years and if she dies first, I don't know what he'll do.

There are many instances of younger men living/loving successfully with much older women.

But as you know, there are many more the other way around. This is because it generally takes men a lot longer to mature emotionally than women, and once they do, they want to go and try it out on a fit young thing. Well, wouldn't you? Luckily for them, many beautiful young women find older men irresistible. And you know what, I don't blame them.

The miracle of the spirit that you see manifest and want in an O has very little to do with his/her chronological age. While it's true that the more times you've been around the sun the more wisdom you're able to access and express, you've got to have it in the first place. The annual orbiting of the sun (every four seasons) just makes it richer. But the meeting of spirits that hits you in the heart and soul can come at any age for both you and O.

Whether you're going to give yourself a heart attack keeping up with your far younger O, or not, is a different matter.

Living with the moon

You think I'm so good at living with other people I can live with the moon now as well?

No, simply be aware of the moon cycle. Make a note of when it's waxing and waning. Make a note of new moon and full moon dates. Use this as a way to gauge your/O's menstrual cycle. Note whether your period comes near the full moon or not. Use that as a rough gauge to estimate ovulation time, which (very) roughly falls at the opposite side of the lunar cycle to the period (funnily enough).

Also be aware that owing to the moon's gravitational pull on your body fluids being far stronger on and around the full moon, you tend to be more mentally unbalanced at that time, i.e., loony (from *la lune*) and therefore more likely to engage in reckless acts of passion you may later regret.

Wishing on an orgasm
(white magic)

Taoist magicians say that whatever you think about as you orgasm will manifest.

As you come, make a wish, i.e., visualize with emotional intensity something you want, or want to occur.

This is powerful manifestation magic because your wish/visualization is supported on its journey by an explosion of the most creative force known to humankind.

This secret, common to Taoist, Tantric, and Western occult systems is popularly known as "sex magic." As such, it can be used in a "right-handed," white magic way or "left-handed," black magic way. The difference is in how you construct your wish/visualization.

The right-handed way is to visualize the essence of what you want happening. So if, for example, you want to have a beautiful love affair, you visualize/wish yourself to be feeling the exact feelings you'd feel when having that love affair, i.e., warm, nurtured, cared for, caring, exhilarated to be alive, and so on.

The left-handed way is to visualize/wish for a precise form to be manifest. So you'd visualize Mary Beth/Nick Angelou being your lover (with or without his/her consent).

Neither is right or wrong, but both have consequences, because according to the immutable laws of cause and effect, the energy you put out comes back to you multiplied.

Taking the right-handed path will bring you the love affair that affords you the essence/feelings you want/need, in the form of the most appropriate lover for you, according to the Tao of the situation.

Taking the left-hand path may bring you Mary/Nick, but because you sent out entrapment energy, you'll land yourself in a trap with Mary/Nick, from which you may find it difficult to extricate yourself one day.

In other words, pay attention to what/who you think about, i.e., wish for, at the moment you hit the peak of the orgasm, because you'll probably get what you want.

Avoiding the pitfalls of practicing alone and falling in love with yourself

Get out more.

Cyber-sex

You may as well get used to it. It's the way things are going. Soon you'll be able to program your computer with your own personal thrust patterns, Big Squeeze preferences, Chi Whooshing requirements, and everything you need to simulate your ideal Wayward Taoist romp. Then all you'll have to do is strap yourself in and let the computer do it to you. And you'll be able to interact with the similar program in O's computer at the same time, so you can synchronize or sabotage each other's movement patterns. Then you'll be able to have a nice cozy chat about it all in your own personal chat room. It won't be long before you can implant a chip into your brain and get the whole thing done while you're asleep, just like when you're dreaming, without eating into your busy schedule. Or maybe we'll be living in caves. Who can tell?

The perils of prolonged wind retention and other gross matters

Avoid the temptation to hold on to a fart in bed, or any time during the sexual dance. Although everyone does it from time to time, if you wish to prevent the possibility of stomach cramps, irritable bowel, and worse, simply excuse yourself and go to the bathroom. But don't come back into the room too soon or you may well bring the fart back in with you.

An old Wayward Taoist ditty goes, "Whether in church, whether in chapel, always let your wind rattle. It makes no difference where ye be, always let your wind go free."

The nonsense of breaking people's hearts

You can't break someone's heart by leaving him/her, even if you promised a thousand and eight times you never would. Even if that person loves you more than the sky loves the sun, moon, and stars themselves.

The way to break a heart is to take a sledgehammer and pound it ferociously and remorselessly a few times.

Hearts don't break from Os leaving. They get stretched, often out of all recognized shape, but they don't break. They're more resilient than that.

In any case, if you give your heart to O to break, it serves you right. Why entrust such a valuable part of yourself to the vagaries, clumsiness, and capriciousness of someone else, who probably doesn't even know how to take care of his/her own heart, let alone yours.

Just like when you nag or tell O off, you give O your words, not your mouth. Give O your love, not your heart.

How to avoid unnecessary aggravation

Don't have sex or speak to anyone for the rest of your life.

Taking one's leave graciously

So how was it for you?

Hard to say. How was it for you?

How was it for me? It's been intense.

In fact, it feels kind of strange getting up off the bed and leaving you here like this.

You see, I've found it hard to say this up till now, but I think I love you.

Thing is though, I've got to go now. I've got things to do, people to heal, books to write, that kind of thing.

Don't take it personally. I'm just busy, that's all.

Look, I'm sure this isn't the last you'll be seeing of me.

I'll be in touch, I really will.

But before I go, some parting words.

If it's a choice of being generous or mean with your sex, be generous.

Whenever you feel you and O are losing your way, stay with the love and the rest will take care of itself.

If you're traumatized into celibacy by the sex = death equation, stop it.

Always identify with what you love in an O.

The Hollywood musicals are all nonsense.

All is fair/unfair in love and war.

About pretty girls: my enlightened friend Russell-the-Spiritual-Firefighter's wise old grandma once told him, "A pretty girl thinks she's got the crown jewels stuffed up her fanny. But when you get to my age, it just looks like a dead pig's eye." In other words, all forms change over time. Rather than identifying with O's physical form, identify instead with his/her unchanging (immortal) spirit.

The Tao for you is the Tao you do. (And vice versa.)

And finally, in the immortal words of Douglas Adams: "So long, and thanks for all the fish."

That's me, I'm spent.

Catchya later, baby. (Don't go changing, now.)

Love (you),

That Crazy B. Doc.

THANK-YOUS

Thanks to everyone who helped make the research, writing, and early postproduction phases of *Barefoot Doctor's Handbook for Modern Lovers* so enjoyable and fulfilling:

Special thanks to Lauren Marino and Cate Tynan for their hand across the transatlantic bridge—the great spirit will reward you in unquantifiable measure (rumor has it).

Judy Piatkus @ Piatkus, publisher, and everyone @ Piatkus, especially including Sandra Rigby, Jana Sommerlad, Philip Cotterell, and Gill Bailey; and most especially Mel Harrison for all her help with the sticky bits.

Michael Alcock @ Michael Alcock Management, literary agent.

Kary Stewart aka Chi Ka @ Ig-nite PR/Ig-nite Radio, PR/media adviser/Twisted Fable facilitator/Clive Alive @ Ig-nite—anchorman.

Carlos Fandango @ Ig-nite and Elsewhere, DJ/PR/soundtrack producer. Soul-Jam coconspirator.

Craig Newman aka the Baron @ Mediator, extreme background mediator.

Sally Clarke @ Mediator, mediator, messenger.

Joe Russell, sounding board/philosophical adviser.

Jake Russell, sounding board/ethical adviser.

Spike Russell, supportive energy dispenser.

Jamie Catto, inspiration facilitator/textual shit-sifting facilitator/creative adviser.

Jessica Howie, textual female-sensibility adviser.

Jane Duval, sounding board/supportive energy dispenser, daisy love science adviser.

Jonty Champelovier, supportive energy dispenser/graphic design adviser *and* facilitator.

Kate Spicer, literary adviser/supportive (inflammable) energy dispenser.

Niel Spencer, astrological adviser.

Zippi-the-Soothsayer, psychic adviser/spell-clearance facilitator.

Karena Callen aka Surge (Supra-Urban/Rural-Goddess-Embodiment), beauty adviser/longevity-continuity-healing balm facilitator.

Bill Reid, illustration realization facilitator.

Dave Anderson, facilitator of Tai Chi @ New PhD and TV.

Ralph-the-Secret-Wizard, show reel facilitator.

Raja Ram, life adviser/spoken word facilitator/supportive energy dispenser.

Dan Harrison, Web site designer/soundtrack composer.

Bérengère, illustrator/dust-therapy facilitator.

Vanessa Kramer, space facilitator/personal development adviser.

Sam Kramer, Ex-Frank-Kramer facilitator/commonsense adviser.

Walter, canine representative.

Lucinda Chambers, fashionability facilitator.

Simon Crow, current affairs/spiritual adviser/concerned energy dispenser.

Shirley Russell, maternal adviser/personage facilitator.

Victor Russell, paternal adviser/personage facilitator.

Lisa Mass, perspective counselor.

Roya Arab, life specialist/morning cake facilitator (that really takes the cake).

Arab Family in general: respect.

Jenny Dyson, magical myth facilitator.

Millie Kendal, chi (qi) background scent adviser.

Fiona Scutt, aka Lady Nada-Och Lassie supervisor.

Anna Bluman, travel adviser.

Richard Cannon, seclusion tour guide/supportive energy dispenser.

Iben Anderson, seclusion tour guide/supportive energy dispenser.

Master Han, chi-activation facilitator.

Gerry Cannon, comedy show host.

Mary Cannon, traditional health adviser.

Jo Simons, volubility facilitator/homeopathic adviser.

Meena Krishnamurthy, medical ratification facilitator.

Lisa Stemmer, modern morals adviser.

Danny Jacobsen @ G-d, spiritual continuity adviser.

Ex-Frank Kramer @ Undifferentiated Absolute, extradimensional facilitator.

Ex-Ronnie Laing @ Distinguished Ontological Spheres, extradimensional supervisor.

Rowan O'Niel @ Witch of America, spell facilitator.

Heidi Easton @ Fittest Woman to Win a BAFTA, aesthetic standards regulating facilitator.

Johnny Toobad @ Popping Up All Over the Place, northeast adviser/facilitator.

Mark @ Newcastle, northern exposure facilitator.

Betsy Rapoport @ Times Books, New York City, Barefoot Doctor Takes America Gently from Behind campaign inspirer.

John-John @ Dominics and BDHQ, vibrational uplift facilitator.

Lara Baum-n @ Strange Romance Inc., aesthetics-uplift facilitator/"havin' words" coconspirator.

Robbie Bear @ Kriya Paradise, vibrational intensification facilitator.

Mother Mary and Baby Jesus aka What-a-Team @ They Don't Make Archetypes Like That These Days, encouragement facilitators.

Stevo Nakovitch @ Alter Ego, fictitious character manifestation facilitator/life adviser.

Nico Ramuda aka Antony Sommers @ The Highgate Egg, Wayward Taoism continuity conspirator.

A general thanks to everyone who helped with research over the years. (What, you think I'm going to mention names?)

A specific thanks to the Wayward Tao, existence/nonexistence facilitator, Source.

A special thanks to you, reader, for reading.

And finally, a big shout to me, author, for being positively charming to work with throughout all the various valleys and peaks of the entire creative process, cheers (you crazy bastard).

Visit Barefoot Doctor's Web site @ www.barefootdoctor/global.com

INDEX

abuse, 223–25
acid, 227–28
acting out desire, 52–53
addiction, 233–34
affirmations, 62
age differences, 234–35
alchemy, inner, 124–27
alcohol, 227
anal sex, 133, 193–94
  licking, 159, 161–62
  Toe in the Hole, 154
  worshiping ass, 159–62
ancestral chi, 131–32
ankles, stroking with toes, 153–54
aphrodisiacs, 226
  dishonesty as, 91
  honesty as, 89
appearance:
  attractiveness, 40–41
  vanity, 41
armpits, 148–49
arms:
  elbow creases, 151–52
  wind in the willows, 146–48
ass. See anal sex.
asshole. See anal sex.
attractiveness, 40–41

back, base of spine, 152
balance, 28–29
beauty, 31–32

belly, 170
Big Squeeze, 117–21
  sexual nirvana, 61
  sperm retention, 131–32
birth control, 30, 105–6, 214
biting, 180–81
black magic, 236–37
bladder energy channel, 149
blow jobs, 171–74
bondage, 216–17
boredom, 77
boundaries, 85
bras, removing, 65
breaking hearts, 238–39
breasts, sucking nipples, 156–59
breathing, 112
  breathing together, 113–14
  connecting your Tan Tiens, 197–98
  Scoopin' the Loop, 125–27
  slowing tempo, 112–13
  Whooshing the Chi, 200–2

calves, massaging, 149
cannabis, 227
celibacy, 232
cheeks, zygomatic kisses, 155–56
chemistry, mystery of, 73
chi (energy), 8, 27–28
  Big Squeeze, 119
  inner alchemy, 124–27

kidney energy, 72
and lack of integrity, 95–96
orgasm and, 18–19
Scoopin' the Loop, 125–27
sperm retention, 131–32
Tan Tiens, 49
Whooshing the Chi, 125,
199–202
Yin and Yang, 45
child abuse, 223–25
clitoris:
cunnilingus, 175–76
manual stimulation, 168–70
clothes, taking off, 64–65
cocaine, 227
cock. *See* penis.
cold sex vs. warm sex, 127
commentary, internal, 136–38
commitment, 103
communication, 86–87
honesty, 88
complexes, 209–10
computers, cyber-sex, 237–38
condoms, 43, 104–7, 213–14, 233
confidentiality, 92–93
consciousness, 25–26
sharing, 49–50
cosmetics, 40
cozy sex, 229–30
creation, connecting with mystery
of, 33
cunnilingus, 174–77
soixante-neuf, 177–78
cyber-sex, 237–38

deceit, 99–100, 104–5
denial, 100–1
deodorants, 60
desire:
acting out vs. containment, 52–53

nature of, 53–55
dick. *See* penis.
dirty sex, 133
discretion, 92–93
dishonesty, 89–90
as an aphrodisiac, 91
distraction, sex as, 231
divorce, 234
drugs, 227–28
dynamics, 74
triangular dynamics, 74, 219–21

ejaculation:
riding the shudders, 190–91
sperm retention, 131–32
sudden surprise ejaculation syndrome (SSES), 71–73, 215
elbow creases, 151–52
embarrassment, 123
energy. *See* chi.
energy channels:
bladder, 149
heart, 148
erection. *See* penis.
erogenous zones, 107–8
eroticism, 50–52
exercise, 64, 110–11
exhibitionism, 221
expectations, 76–77
eyes open vs. eyes closed, 133–34

face, zygomatic kisses, 155–56
fairness, 101–2
faithfulness, 96–97
faking orgasm, 109
falling in love, 93–95
fantasies, 56–58
acting out, 129
soul mates, 76
farting, 238

feet:
augmenting coital stimulation
with, 194–95
Gateway to the Soul, 145–46
stroking with toes, 153–54
sucking toes, 152–53
Toe in the Hole, 154
fetishes, 43
fidelity, 96–97
fingers:
between the fingers, 151
knuckles, 150
stimulating vagina with, 178–79
fitness, physical, 64, 110–11
flexibility, 64, 110
flirting, 82–83
floating harem, 81–82
forearm, wind in the willows,
146–47
four ounces of pressure, 116–17
French kisses, 161–64
friends, 102–3, 233
frigidity, 210
full-power pumping, 191–92

Gate of Mortality, 118–19
Gateway to the Soul, 145–46
gay men, 12
genitals, size, 90–91
grinding, 194

hands:
augmenting coital stimulation
with, 194–95
between the fingers, 151
clitoral stimulation, 168–70
hand jobs, 164–67
knuckles, 150
stimulating vagina with, 178–79
harem, floating, 81–82

heart energy channel, 148
heart-to-heart connection, 154–55
hearts, breaking, 238–39
hepatitis, 105
heroin, 228
herpes, 105
hips, relaxing, 115
HIV, 105
homosexuality, 12
honesty, 88
as aphrodisiac, 89
dishonesty, 89–90
dishonesty as an aphrodisiac,
91
hookers, 218–19
hygiene, 41–42, 232
anal sex, 160, 161–62, 193

Immortal Spirit Body, 46–47
impotence, 211–13
incest, 222–23
inhibitions, 63
inner alchemy, 124–27
insight, 88
integrity, 95–96
intensifying sexual tension, 111
internal commentary, 136–38
interpersonal space, 85

jade pillow, supporting, 146
jealousy, 229
jerking off
hand jobs, 164–67
See also masturbation.
jing, 131–32

ketamine, 228
kidney energy:
ancestral chi, 131
impotence, 211

sudden surprise ejaculation
   syndrome (SSES), 72, 215
kissing:
   French kisses, 162–64
   zygomatic kisses, 155–56
knees, back of, 149–50
knuckles, 150
kundalini-yoga, 110

lazy sex, 229–30
legs:
   back of knees, 149–50
   calves, 149
lesbians, 12
libido, fluctuating levels, 231
love, 29–30, 46
   falling in love, 93–95
   fidelity, 96–97
   sex as an expression of, 4–5
   sexual love, 30
love bites, 181
lubricants, 226
lying, 89–90, 100–1

magic, wishing on an orgasm,
   236–37
"magpie bridge," 125–26
manners, 92–93
marriage, 217, 234
martial arts, 110
massage, 231
   calves, 149
   Gateway to the Soul, 145–46
masturbation, 129–31
   being comfortable with your sex-
      uality, 61
   fantasies, 57–58
MDMA, 228
meditation, counting repetitions,
   70

menstrual cycle, 73, 235
meridians, chi, 28
monogamy:
   nonserial, 80
   serial, 77–79, 82
moon cycle, 235–36
moral codes, 35–36
mouth:
   augmenting coital stimulation
      with, 194–95
   blow jobs, 171–74
   cunnilingus, 174–78
   soixante-neuf, 177–78
movement, 66
   tempo, 68–69
mystery:
   of chemistry, 73
   of creation, 33

nakedness, 64–65
navel, 170
neck, supporting the jade pillow,
   146
nipping, 181
nipples, sucking, 156–59
nirvana:
   sexual, 67–68
   sperm retention, 132
   Whooshing the Chi, 202–3
Ni Wan Peaks, 67

oral sex:
   blow jobs, 171–74
   cunnilingus, 174–78
   soixante-neuf, 177–78
orgasm, 121–22
   afterward, 203–4
   Big Squeeze, 117–21
   blow jobs, 174
   cunnilingus, 176

energy flow and, 19
feigning, 109
inability to reach, 216
perfect fuck, 141
play in your mind, 80
responsibility for, 122
sexual nirvana, 67–68
sperm retention, 131–32
sudden surprise ejaculation syndrome (SSES), 71–72, 215
wishing on, 236–37
orgies, 220–21
ovulation, 73, 235

pain, sadomasochism, 216
passion, nature of, 55–56
penis:
blow jobs, 171–74
condoms, 106–7
entering vagina, 187
grinding, 194
hand jobs, 164–67
impotence, 211–13
riding the shudders, 190–91
Sexual Stillpoint, 191
size, 90–91
thrusting, 188–90
perfect fuck, 139–41
perfect mate, 76
performance, sex as, 43–44
perineum:
Big Squeeze, 118–21
riding the shudders, 190–92
periods, 235
personal space, 85
perversion, 216–17
pheromones, 59, 60
physical fitness, 64, 110
pinching, 181–82
planning the moment, 128–29

play in your mind, 79–80
falling in love, 94–95
polyandry, 81
polygamy, 81, 82
polygyny, 81
pornography, 229
positions, 114–15, 183–85
moving between, 185–87
possessiveness, 94, 96, 228–29
power-yoga, 110
pregnancy:
preventing, 105, 214
sex after, 234
sex during, 234
premature ejaculation, 70–73, 215
pressure, four ounces of, 116–17
problems, 207–8
procreational sex, 30–31
promiscuity, 233–34
props, 43
prostitution, 218–19
pubic pinch, 155
pumping, full-power, 191–92
pure sexual intelligence, 56–57
pussy. See vagina.

rape, 208–9
recreational sex, 30–31
Reich, Wilhelm, 18
relationships:
age differences, 234–35
boundaries and personal/
interpersonal space, 85
breaking hearts, 238–39
chemistry, 73
commitment, 103
communication, 86–87
deceit, 99–100, 104–5
dishonesty, 89–91
dynamics, 74

falling in love, 93–95
fidelity, 96–97
floating harem, 81–82
friends, 102–3
honesty, 88
illusion of, 37–38
loyalty, 97
manners, 92–93
monogamy, 77–80
perfect mate, 76
soul mates, 75
treachery, 97–98
trust, 85–86
relaxation, 115–16
repetitions, counting, 70
responsibility, 92, 122
riding the shudders, 190–91
rude, 63

sadomasochism, 216–17
saliva, French kiss, 163–64
scent, 42, 60
Scoopin' the Loop, 125–27, 200
scratching, 179–80
seduction, 84–85
self-consciousness, 41
self-esteem, 61–63, 83
serial monogamy, 77–79, 82
sex addiction, 233
sexiness, 38–40
sex magic, 236–37
sex parties, 221
sex toys, 225
sexual intelligence, 56–58
sexuality, being comfortable with
  your, 60–61
sexual love, 30
sexual nirvana, 67–68
  sperm retention, 131–32
  Whooshing the Chi, 202–3

sexual problems, 207–8
Sexual Stillpoint, 191
sexual tension, intensifying, 111
sexually transmitted diseases
  (STDs), 58, 105, 213–14
signals, alertness to, 69
size, genitals, 90–91
smells, 42, 59–60
soap, 60
socks, removing, 65
soixante-neuf, 177–78
Soul, Gateway to the, 145–46
soul mates, 75
sounds:
  vocalizing during sex, 122–24
  voice, 86–87
so what? factor, 141
space, interpersonal, 85
sperm retention, 131–32
spine, base of, 152
Spirit Body, 46–47
spiritualizing sex, 8–9, 22–24
stamina, 64, 110
Stillpoint, Sexual, 191
stopping when you want,
  134–36
strangers, sex with, 103–4, 233
stress relief, sex as, 231
sudden surprise ejaculation
  syndrome (SSES), 71–73, 215
suppleness, 64, 110

tai chi, 110
Tan Tiens (TTs), 47–49, 196,
  197–98
Tantric sex, 23
Tao, 24–27
Taoism, 20–22, 23–24
teasing, 111, 135
techniques, integrating, 138

tempo, 68–69
  alternating rhythms, 192
  slowing breath tempo, 112–13
tension:
  intensifying sexual, 111
  relaxing, 115–16
The Erotic Moment (TEM),
  50–52
threesomes, 219–21
Three Tan Tiens (TTTs), 47–49,
  196, 197–98
thrush, 105
tickling, 182–83
toes:
  stroking with, 153–54
  sucking, 152–53
  Toe in the Hole, 154
tongue:
  blow jobs, 171–74
  cunnilingus, 175–76
  French kiss, 162–64
touch, four ounces of pressure,
  116–17
toys, 225
transcendental aspects, 195–97
treachery, 97–98
triangular dynamics, 74, 219–21
trust, 85–86
  fidelity, 96–97

undressing, 64–65

vagina:
  cunnilingus, 174–78

putting two fingers up, 178–79
sacred entry, 187–88
Sexual Stillpoint, 191
size, 90
thrusts, 188–90
vaginismus, 210–11
vanity, 41
vibrators, 225
visualization, wishing on an
  orgasm, 236–37
voice:
  communication, 86–87
  vocalizing during sex, 122–24
voyeurism, 221

Warm sex vs. cold sex, 127
white magic, 236–37
Whooshing the Chi, 125, 199–203
willy. See penis.
wind in the willows, 146–48
wind retention, 238
wishing on an orgasm, 236–37
womb, 169–70
Wu Wei, 128

Yin and Yang, 26–27
  breathing together, 113–14
  eternal dance, 44–45
  perfect mate, 76
  Scoopin' the Loop, 125
  soixante-neuf, 177–78
yoga, 110

zygomatic kisses, 155–56

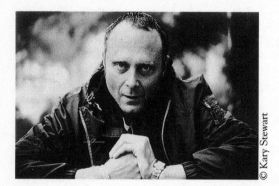

© Kary Stewart

Stephen Russell is a healer, acupuncturist, martial arts teacher, musician, performance artist, and writer. One of the leading gurus for global youth culture, he writes for *Lotus* magazine and is the alternative health columnist for *The Observer* (London). He has penned another book in the Handbook Series, *Barefoot Doctor's Guide to the Tao*, as well as *The Tao of Sexual Massage*, which has sold over 500,000 copies worldwide. Reachable at www.barefootdoctorglobal.com, he lives in London, New Mexico, and Thailand.